617.462 BLA (M)

D0301654

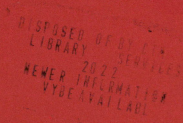

DISPOSED OF BY CTM
LIBRARY SERVICES
2022
NEWER INFORMATION
MAYBE AVAILABLE

PC00002617

TRANSURETHRAL RESECTION

Fourth Edition

J P Blandy CBE, DM, MCh, FRCS, FACS, FRCSI (Hon)
Emeritus Professor of Urology, The Royal London Hospital and
Medical College; Consulting Urologist, St Peter's Hospital, UK

and

R G Notley MS, FRCS
Consultant Urological Surgeon, The Royal Surrey Hospital,
Guildford, UK

I S I S
MEDICAL
M E D I A

Oxford

First published by Pitman Medical Publishing Co Ltd, 1971
Second edition, 1978
Third edition by Butterworth-Heinemann Ltd, 1993
Fourth edition by Isis Medical Media Ltd, 1998

British Library Cataloguing in Publication Data.
A catalogue record for this title is available from
the British Library

ISBN 1 899066 84 5

Blandy, J P (John)
Transurethral resection (4th revised edition)
John Blandy and Richard Notley

Always refer to the manufacturer's Prescribing
Information before prescribing drugs cited in this book.

Typeset by
Creative Associates, Oxford

Reproduction by
Create Publishing Services, Bath

Produced by Phoenix Offset, HK
Printed in China

Distributed in the USA by
Mosby-Year Book, Inc, 11830 Westline Industrial Drive
St Louis MO63145, USA

Distributed in the rest of the world by
Oxford University Press, Saxon Way West, Corby
Northamptonshire NN18 9ES, UK

Contents

Preface

From the Preface to the first edition (1971)

'Alas, the prevailing climate of surgical opinion is still against transurethral resection, largely, I believe, because it does not understand what the operation is supposed to be doing. How often, for instance, does one still hear it said that TUR is only suitable for the small fibrous gland or the carcinoma? How often is it implied that a transurethral resection is in some way less thorough than an open prostatectomy, and so generally has to be done again? Both these notions are false. The real objection to TUR is that it is so hard to learn and so hard to teach. The object of this book is to make it slightly less hard.'

Preface to the fourth edition

When those words were written, transurethral resection (TUR) was, at least in Europe, not quite respectable. Transvesical or retropubic prostatectomy was the correct treatment for prostatic hypertrophy; open cystodiathermy or partial cystectomy was the standard treatment for anything but the smallest bladder tumour. It is ironic that transurethral resection is today the gold standard against which new methods must be compared. Nevertheless, despite its new respectability, TUR, like any operation in surgery, has to be learned—a difficult process even though it has become immeasurably easier and safer thanks to rod lens, fibre light and television.

We do not aim to deal with any of the wondrous new treatments which appear almost every month, each guaranteed to replace TUR: pills and injections; hyper- and hypo-thermia; focused ultrasound; expanding balloons, wire and plastic stents; lasers and roly-balls which coagulate or vapourize the prostate; TVP, TULIP, TUNA, TUNIP, TUVP, TUMT, and all the other acronyms that dash across the urological scene like clouds in summer.

No doubt one day some such new method will supplant TUR—for it is by no means perfect. Until then young urologists must learn transurethral resection and must learn to do it right. This book, whose practical tips have all been learned the hard way, is for them.

J.P.B. and R.G.N.

Acknowledgements

The authors wish to thank a number of individuals and firms for their invaluable cooperation in the production of this book. The first of these is Alastair Holdoway of Video South Medical Television for his generous help in a number of ways, but especially with the production of the coloured endoscopic photographs. Rimmer Brothers, Karl Storz Endoscopy (UK) and KeyMed have again been generous in their help with the illustrations of the endoscopic equipment.

Chapter 1
History

The ancients, who thought that the bladder was divided by a horizontal septum, knew little about obstruction at its outflow, though Galen must have divided the prostate and bladder neck regularly when performing lateral lithotomy[1]. Oribasius of Pergamum, writing his synopsis at the command of the Emperor Julian in the fourth century AD, proposed to cut through the prostate by a perineal incision in cases of retention of urine where it was impossible to pass a catheter, considering that the risk of fistula after this operation was preferable to death from unrelieved retention. Ambroise Paré seems to have been aware of the entity of bladder neck obstruction, and devised catheters with a sharp cutting cup at the tip with which pieces of the bladder neck could be torn away (Fig. 1.1). Morgagni, Valsalva and Bartholin all wrote on the subject[1-3], but it was John Hunter who demonstrated, in a series of specimens, the progressive effects and complications of prostatic obstruction. One of these was a classic example of obstruction by enlargement of the middle lobe[4] which his brother-in-law Everard Home subsequently published and claimed as his own original observation — plagiary soon denounced by his contemporaries[5] (Fig. 1.2).

As for treatment, there was only the catheter and men were admitted to hospital to be 'schooled' in how to pass it. Even at the end of the nineteenth century the mortality of catheterization was still as high as 20% in the first six months[6].

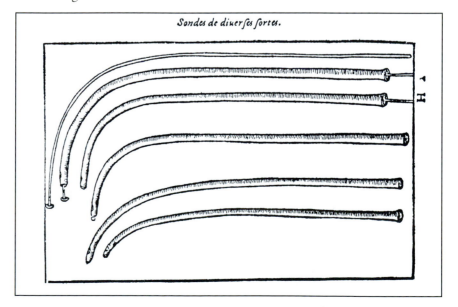

Figure 1.1
Catheters armed with cups for removing 'carnosities' from the urethra and possibly also the bladder neck. Ambroise Paré 1510–1590.

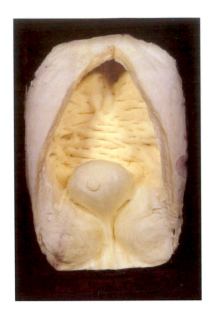

Figure 1.2
John Hunter's specimen showing a large middle lobe. Courtesy of the Trustees of the Hunterian Museum, The Royal College of Surgeons of England.

Probably the first surgeon to attempt an open division of the bladder neck was Sir William Blizard in about 1806 (Fig. 1.3) who described a patient in the London Hospital who lay with an indwelling catheter and subsequently died with an abscess in each lateral lobe of the prostate[5]. Blizard reflected that:

This person might have been successfully treated by dividing the prostate with a double gorget cutting on both sides introduced in the usual way on a staff into the bladder. It would have relieved the immediate distress, and might have laid the foundation for a cure. This is not a speculative remark. I have several times performed such an operation in cases of disease of the prostate gland which I have thought within its scope of relief, with complete success.

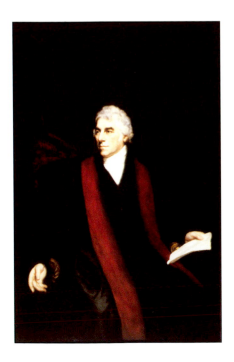
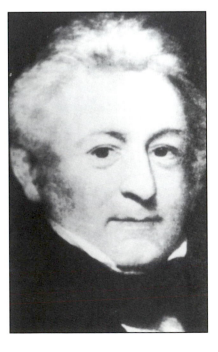

Figure 1.3 (left)
Sir William Blizard. Courtesy of the President and Council of the Royal College of Surgeons of England.

Figure 1.4 (right)
Sir George James Guthrie. Courtesy of the President and Council of the Royal College of Surgeons of England.

Of Blizard's contemporaries, Guthrie (Fig. 1.4) at the Westminster Hospital, with an international reputation for the conservative treatment of limb wounds before and after Waterloo, noted the role of the bladder neck in outflow obstruction:

> No greater error has been committed in surgery than that which supposes the third lobe, as it is called, of the prostate to be the common cause of those difficulties in making water which occur so frequently in elderly people and sometimes in young ones. I do not deny that a portion of the prostate does enlarge and project into the bladder, preventing the flow of urine from it; but I mean to affirm that this evil takes place more frequently, and is more effectually caused by, disease of the neck of the bladder, totally unconnected with the prostate, than by disease of that part[5].

Understanding the nature of the 'bar at the neck of the bladder', Guthrie devised a means of dividing it which would be less traumatic than Blizard's perineal incision. He ordered a sound to be made for him with a concealed knife which could be projected to cut through the 'bar, dam or stricture' without injuring the adjacent parts (Fig. 1.5). It is often said that Guthrie had in mind the kind of bladder neck stenosis which may occur without enlargement of the prostate, but in his illustration (Fig. 1.6) of a specimen lent him by Goldwyer Andrews, Blizard's colleague and successor at the London Hospital, it is clear that he was thinking of typical middle lobe enlargement, and the concealed knife was intended to cut the ring of bladder muscle that imprisons and traps the adenoma.

Concealed knives similar to that of Guthrie were later devised by Civiale and Mercier[7] (Fig 1.7). Mercier claimed to have done 300 successful operations—a figure doubted by Guyon[8]. Years later, when Hugh Hampton Young devised his punch, he generously gave credit and priority to Mercier[9].

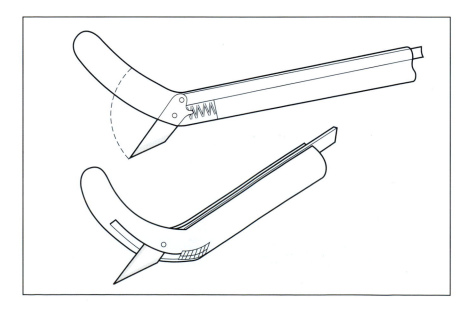

Figure 1.5
Guthrie's concealed knife, based on his description.

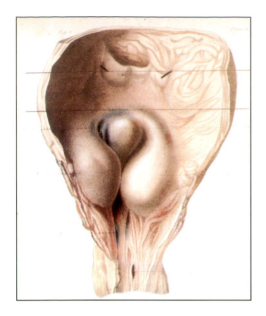

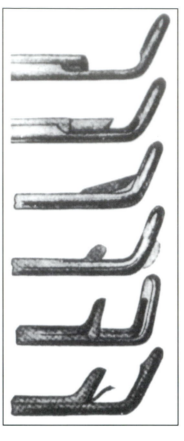

Figure 1.6 (left)
Guthrie's prostate specimen, supplied to him by Golwyer Andrews of The London Hospital.

Figure 1.7 (right)
Concealed knives devised by Civiale and Mercier.

Inevitably any kind of incision or cold punch resection was more or less blind and bloody: to overcome these defects surgery had to wait for the application of electrical engineering to urology. The first step was taken by Bottini[10] who devised an instrument like a lithotrite whose male blade was heated by direct current to burn a channel through the neck of the bladder (Fig. 1.8). There was no bleeding until the slough came away, but it was still blind, and it was difficult to know exactly which tissues were being burnt. Bottini claimed to have done 57 cases with two deaths and 12 failures[10].

Bottini's work was taken up by his contemporaries. Fenwick (Fig. 1.9), Chetwood and Wishard all attempted to improve Bottini's instrument, but the results were unimpressive[11–13]. 'No permanent good ever came of it', wrote Reginald Harrison of St Peter's Hospital[14] who preferred to open the bladder or perform urethrotomy so as to be able to dilate the internal meatus with his finger. If the patient were unfit for either of these procedures, then

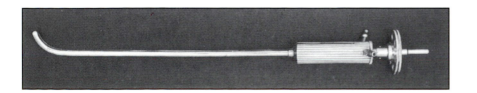

Figure 1.8
Bottini's instrument for heating the prostate. Courtesy of the Institute of Urology.

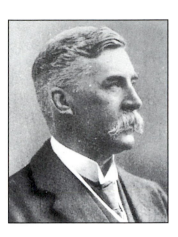

Figure 1.9
Edwin Hurry Fenwick.

he was to be given a permanent suprapubic tube of the improved pattern then being introduced by Buckston Browne[14].

At the end of the nineteenth century the standard treatment at St Peter's Hospital was still 'catheter schooling', supplemented by vasectomy (since this was believed to lead to testicular atrophy, and in turn to shrinkage of the prostate[6]). Looking back on these years, Frank Kidd[15] noted that up to 8% of men treated in this way would be dead of uraemia or infection within a month.

It was in this climate that enucleative prostatectomy by the suprapubic or perineal route was introduced[7]. First recorded at St Bartholomew's Hospital in 1884[16] it was independently developed by Goodfellow in Tombstone, Arizona (1885)[17], McGill in Leeds (1887)[18], Mansell-Moullin at the London Hospital (1892)[19], Fuller in New York (1895)[20] and Freyer at St Peter's (1900)[21] (Fig. 1.10). Thanks very largely to Freyer's enthusiasm and energy the transvesical or Freyer operation soon overtook all other forms of treatment, but even the pioneers in the field were concerned that the amount of tissue removed 'is often so small that it seems ridiculous to have to perform suprapubic operation for its removal'[22].

It was this concern which led Hugh Hampton Young, one of the pioneers of perineal prostatectomy, to look again at Mercier's concept of using a sharp tubular knife, like a cork-borer (Fig. 1.11).

Figure 1.10
Sir Peter Freyer.

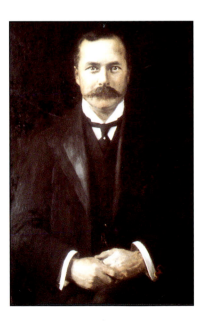

Figure 1.11
Hugh Hampton Young's punch.

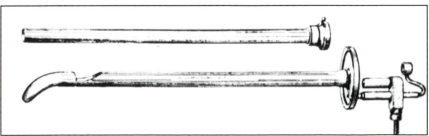

'I called my instrument a prostatic excisor and the operation excision. The internes promptly dubbed the instrument 'the punch'[22]. The first punch was very simple and without any means of haemostasis: this was only possible thanks to the development of diathermy[23].

Soon after the discovery that very high-frequency alternating current did not excite nerve or muscle, the heating effect at the site of contact would be used to cauterize warts on the skin, and by 1910 Beer was using the same current through a cystoscope to cauterize 'warts' in the bladder[24]. The electric cystoscope, pioneered in Germany by Nitze, and introduced to the UK by Fenwick, was now in general use, although it had taken Fenwick a decade to overcome the early prejudice against it. Fenwick was once laughed off the rostrum at the Medical Society of London for suggesting that the electric cystoscope was anything more than a gimmick, since every proper surgeon knew that the right way to explore the bladder was with a finger introduced via the perineum[25].

With the early operating cystoscopes and the early spark-gap diathermy machines one could produce a controlled Bottini burn at the neck of the bladder, although it took a series of sittings before a sufficiently large channel could be burned away. This method was developed in New York by Stevens[26] and Bugbee[27], and in France by Luys[7,28] (Fig. 1.12).

Young's approach was far more bold: he tried to cut away the tissue, and then stop the bleeding with the diathermy (Fig. 1.13). This combination of the cold punch with diathermy haemostasis was rapidly developed by Young, Braasch, Bumpus and Caulk[29] until by 1930 Caulk reported that he could resect 85% of his cases with the punch, and had only one death in 510 cases[30]. The 'cold punch' had arrived. It did however have a major drawback: the surgeon's view was obscured just as the tissue was being cut off, and this made it difficult and even dangerous to use.

A different principle was being developed at the same time, using a hot wire to cut through the tissue. As early as 1895 Fenwick[11] had

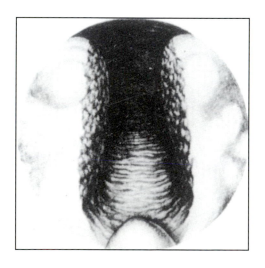

Figure 1.12
'Forage' of the prostate.
From Luys (1935)[28].

Figure 1.13
Gershom Thomson's combination diathermy and punch. Courtesy of the Institute of Urology.

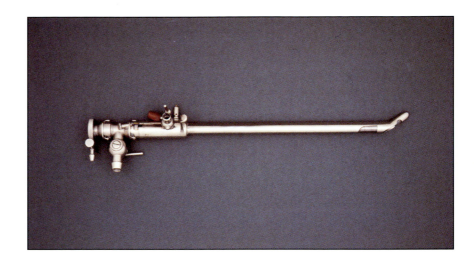

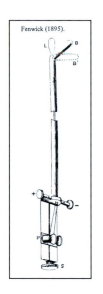

Fenwick (1895).

Figure 1.14
Fenwick's 'galvanic écraseur'.

designed a 'galvanic ecraseur' with a wire snare, heated white hot, to cut through the projecting parts of the middle lobe (Fig. 1.14). In practice it is difficult to cut through the prostate with a hot wire: it drags, sticks and carbonizes. Loop resection was not a practical possibility until 1926 when Maximilian Stern[31] tried out the new powerful radio-frequency valve diathermy machine invented by Wappler. Stern described how this more powerful current would create 'a luminous ring or halo which causes eruption of cells in its path as the loop is advanced, leaving no carbonized tissue either on the loop or the cut surface of the gutter it leaves in the tissues'[31]. It may not have carbonized the tissue, but neither did it stop the bleeding. For a time urologists would use two machines: Wappler's new valve 'endotherm' for cutting, and the old-fashioned spark-gap diathermy for haemostasis. Eventually, enterprising manufacturers supplied both circuits in one box with variable current outputs that allowed the surgeon to cut or coagulate as necessary.

To Stern's diathermy system was soon added the 'foroblique' telescope devised by McCarthy, and the combination became the Stern-McCarthy resectoscope, a sturdy and reliable instrument, which is the prototype of all the present-day instruments (Fig. 1.15).

By 1930 hot-wire or cold-punch instruments were available to any surgeon who would take the trouble to learn how to use them. At first the aim was limited, to cut a groove through the middle lobe, or to excise small glands and little fibrous bladder necks where there were only 5 or 10 g of tissue to be taken away.

It was in the Middle West that transurethral surgery really grew up. By 1936 Thomson and Buchtel of the Mayo Clinic[32] reported 200 cases from whom they had removed more than 20 g of tissue. Five years later in Minneapolis Creevy did not consider a prostate 'large' unless he had removed more than 30 g[33] and it was not long before the concept of transurethral resection had been entirely changed. No longer was it the intention to perform a kind of forage of the gland, but to remove the adenoma right down to the capsule

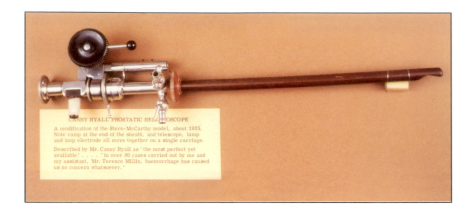

in a way that was no less complete and no less thorough than that of the surgeon's finger at transvesical prostatectomy.

Detailed accounts of how to perform a complete transurethral prostatectomy were published in 1943 by Reed Nesbit of Ann Arbor[34] and Roger Barnes[35] of Los Angeles, but by now the Second World War was raging and at least in Europe there were other matters to occupy the attention of surgeons, and there was a hiatus in the development of transurethral surgery.

Between the wars, transurethral resection using the cold punch had been taken up with enthusiasm by Wardill in Newcastle who, like Lane in Dublin, had been to the Mayo clinic to see for himself[36]. Hot-wire resection had been taken up by Canny Ryall and Terence Millin at All Saints[37,38], Kenneth Walker[39] at St Paul's and Ogier Ward at St Peter's but their efforts were hampered by the unreliability of their diathermy equipment. As Millin was later to confide, 'My personal experiences with TUR commenced in 1930 and by 1949 I had carried out some 2000 TURs. By 1940 my percentage was 80% approximately but with the introduction of safer open prostatectomy the percentage declined to less than 10% in the years before I retired'[40].

One critical factor was that the more powerful diathermy machines were commandeered from hospitals to be used to block enemy radar[41] and even 10 years later few hospitals were equipped with diathermy that would cut under water. The other factor was that, after the war, the returning surgeons were greeted with the news that Millin himself, protagonist of transurethral resection, had almost given it up in favour of the retropubic operation. The new operation was simple, easy to teach, and easy to learn: coupled with the introduction of aseptic measures and the sulphonamides, open prostatectomy became much more safe[42]. The fact that it was still nothing like as safe as transurethral resection was ignored[6]. Even as

Figure 1.16
Harold Hopkins.

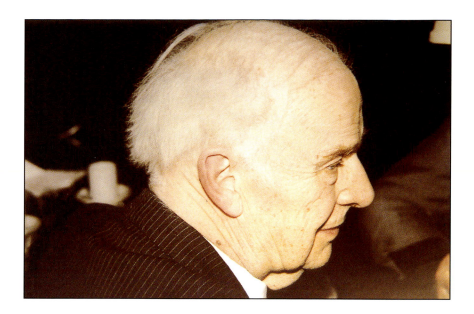

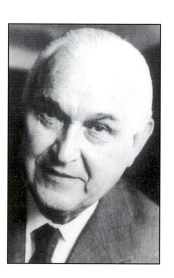

Figure 1.17
Karl Storz.

late as 1960, Salvaris[43] pointed out that in 1200 open operations at St Peter's Hospital the mean weight of prostate was only 42 g. His article was turned down by British journals, and eventually only found its way into print in Australia.

With the exception perhaps of those who were fortunate enough to work in Dublin with Lane[36], any young surgeon who wished to learn transurethral resection had to go to North America. There we encountered a whole new world of astonishing urological expertise. Resection of a 50 g prostate was routine: the bleeding was stopped completely, and patients went home within a few days: what a difference from the grisly procedure with which we were familiar back home. On our return Geoffrey Chisholm, Joe Smith and other converts began to practise and preach what we had learned[36]. But change was slow: there was still a shortage of effective diathermy equipment, the telescopes were dim and the lighting unreliable. The operation continued to be very difficult to teach.

Then came the three inventions of the late Harold Hopkins (Fig. 1.16) which were to change transurethral resection completely. The first was the rod-lens telescope, which owed its development to the imagination and enterprize of Karl Storz (Fig. 1.17). The second was the flexible glass fibre light cable, which provided limitless, unfailing illumination. The third was the coordinated flexible glass cable which made it possible for a pupil to watch the operation.

Thanks to these improvements and to the increasing confidence in transurethral surgery, there crept in another equally important development in urology: transurethral resection of bladder tumours. From the early 1930s small papillary tumours were coagulated with cystoscopic electrodes but when they were too large to be 'fulgurated' it was necessary to open the bladder and remove them with a diathermy snare after which the base was sown with radon seeds or tantalum wire[44]. Today these operations have been completely given up.

These changes have come about entirely due to the advances made in urological instruments. When today we sit down to resect a bladder tumour or a prostate we should remember with gratitude those 'grand originals' who struggled so hard to make it possible[45].

References

1. Murphy LTJ. *The History of Urology*. Springfield: Thomas, 1972.
2. Paré A. *Oevres completes avec figures*. JF Malgaigne (ed.) Paris: Bailliere, 1840.
3. Gutierrez R. *History of Urology* Bransford Lewis (ed.) Vol. 2. Baltimore: Williams and Wilkins, 1933: 137.
4. Palmer JF (ed.) *The Works of John Hunter*. London: Longmans, 1835.
5. Guthrie GJ. *On the Anatomy and Diseases of the Urinary and Sexual Organs*. London: Churchill, 1836.
6. Blandy JP. Surgery of the benign prostate: the first Sir Peter Freyer Memorial Lecture. *J Irish Med Ass* 1977; **70**: 517.
7. Rognon LM, Raymond G. Historique de l'hyperplasie bénigne de la prostate. *Ann Urol* 1992; **26**: 167.
8. Guyon F. *Les prostatiques. Ann des mal des Org Génitourin* 1885; **3**: 328.
9. Young HH. A new procedure (punch operation) for small prostatic bars and contractures of the prostatic orifice. *J Am Med Ass* 1913; **60**: 253.
10. Bottini E. Die galvanocaustische Diaerese zur Radical-Behandlung der Ischurie bei Hypertrophie der Prostata. *Arch Klin Chir* 1897; **54**: 98.
11. Fenwick EH. *Urinary Surgery*. 2nd edn. Bristol: Wright, 1895.
12. Chetwood CH. Contracture of the neck of the bladder. *Med Rec* 1901; **59**: 767.
13. Wishard WN. Notes on surgery of the prostate. *J Cutan Genitourin Dis* 1925; **10**: 105.
14. Harrison R. *Lectures on the Surgical Disorders of the Urinary Organs*. 4th edn. London: Churchill, 1893.
15. Kidd F. *Urinary Surgery: a review*. London: Longmans Green, 1910.
16. St Bartholomew's Hospital Reports. *Statistical Tables* 1885; **21**: 79.
17. Goodfellow G. Prostatectomy in general especially by the perineal route. *J Am Med Ass* 1904; Nov 12: 1448.
18. McGill AF. Suprapubic prostatectomy. *Br Med J* 1887; **2**: 1104.
19. Mansell-Moullin CW. *Enlargement of the Prostate: its treatment and cure*. London: Lewis, 1894.
20. Fuller E. Six successful and successive cases of prostatectomy. *J Cut Genitourin Dis.* 1895; **13**: 229.
21. Freyer PJ. A clinical lecture on total extirpation of the prostate for radical cure of enlargement of that organ. *Br Med J* 1901; **2**: 125.
22. Young HH. Discussion after symposium on resection. *J Urol* 1932; **28**: 585.
23. Nation EF. Evolution of knife-punch resectoscope. *Urology* 1976; **7**: 417.
24. Beer E. Removal of neoplasms of the urinary bladder. A new method employing high frequency (Oudin) currents through a catheterising cystoscope. *J Am Med Ass* 1910; **54**: 1768.
25. Morson C. Personal communication to JPB. 1969.
26. Stevens AR. Value of cauterisation by high frequency current in certain cases of prostatic obstruction. *New York Med J* 1913; **98**: 170.
27. Bugbee HG. The relief of vesical obstruction in selected cases: preliminary report. *New York State Med H* 1913; **13**: 410.
28. Luys G. Traitement de l'hypertrophie de la prostate par la voie endourétrale. *Clinique* 1913; **44**: 693.
29. Collings CW. History of endoscopic surgery. In: Barnes RW (ed.) *Endoscopic Prostatic Surgery*. London: Kimpton, 1943.
30. Caulk JR. Obstructing lesions of the prostate. Influence of the author's cautery punch operation in decreasing the necessity for prostatectomy. *J Am Med Ass* 1930; **94**: 375.
31. Stern M. Resections of obstructions at the vesical orifice. *J Am Med Ass* 1926; **87**: 1726.
32. Thomson GT, Buchtel H. Transurethral resection of the large prostate: a review of 200 cases in which 25 grams or more of tissue was removed. *J Urol* 1936; **36**: 43.
33. Creevy CD. Resection of the 'large' prostate: technic and results. *J Urol* 1941; **45**: 715.

34. Nesbit RM. *Transurethral Prostatectomy*. Baltimore: Thomas, 1943.
35. Barnes RW. *Endoscopic Prostatic Surgery*. London: Kimpton, 1943.
36. Blandy JP, Williams JP. *The History of the British Association of Urological Surgeons 1945–1995*. London: BAUS, 1995.
37. Ryall C, Millin T. An alternative to prostatectomy. *Lancet* 1932; **2**: 121.
38. Ryall C, Millin T. Endoscopic resection of the prostate–a survey. *Urol Cut Rev* 1933; **37**: 52.
39. Walker KM. Perurethral operations for prostatic obstruction. *Br Med J* 1925; **1**: 201.
40. Millin T. Personal communication to JPB. 1969.
41. Jones RV. *Most Secret War*. London: Hamilton, 1978: 126.
42. Wilson Hey H. Asepsis in prostatectomy. *Br J Surg* 1945; **33**: 41.
43. Salvaris M. Retropubic prostatectomy: an evaluation of 1200 operations. *Med J Austral* 1960; **47**: 370.
44. Dix VW, Shanks W, Tresidder GC *et al*. Carcinoma of the bladder: treatment by diathermy snare excision and interstitial irradiation. *Br J Urol* 1970; **42**: 213.
45. Blandy JP. The history of urology in the British Isles. In: Mattelaer JJ (ed.) *De Historia Urologiae Europaeae*, vol. 2: 11–22. European Association of Urology, Kortrijk, 1995.

Chapter 2
The instruments

When a government purchases a modern missile, it speaks in terms of a 'weapons system', implying not only the rockets but all the complex electronic guidance systems and maintenance arrangements that go with them. So, also, with a resectoscope it is wise to think of the entire weapons system: the light source, the diathermy equipment, and the closed circuit television system.

The resectoscope

Several different instrument systems are available today and the trainee should take trouble to use as many different resectoscopes as possible. When purchasing one, especially when it comes to equipping a department, it is even more necessary to think in terms of a 'weapons system'. Bear certain points in mind: all these instruments are very expensive, and all resectoscopes can be made to do good work in the hands of an expert. It is humiliating to recall that 50 years ago the master resectionists of the Middle West were removing 100 g an hour with a filament-lit Stern-McCarthy. An expensive tennis racket does not guarantee victory at Wimbledon. If you do have to use an unfamiliar resectoscope it is no more difficult than adjusting to a new car: you do not have to learn to drive all over again.

Interchangeable equipment

Except for diagnostic flexible cystoscopy, the indications for using a rigid cystoscope nearly always imply that something else will be done. You may need to catheterize a ureter, biopsy a suspicious lesion, resect a tumour, incise a bladder neck, incise a urethral stricture or crush a stone. You must be able to go ahead and do any of these things without having first to fiddle with different light leads and water connections. The first requirement then is for a complete kit of interchangeable instruments.

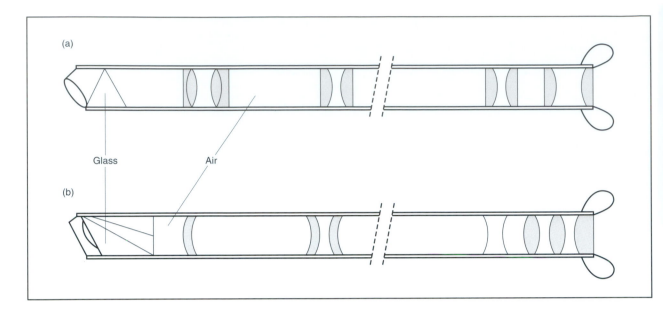

(a)

Glass   Air

(b)

Figure 2.1
(a) Conventional telescope.
(b) Hopkins' rod lens
*   telescope.*

Service

The instrument system you finally choose will depend on several factors. First will be the amount of money you or your hospital can afford: but no less important should be the question of after-sales service. You must be able to get rapid and efficient service from a manufacturer's agent who has a representative in your own city, who visits your hospital regularly, knows you and your operating theatre team, and has won a reputation for promptness and reliability. It is no good buying a Rolls-Royce if their nearest agent is in Ruritania.

Spares

Make sure you have an adequate number of spare parts. It is reckless to embark on a resection and be held up because the lamp in the light source has blown and there is no spare; because water has got into the telescope and you can no longer see; because the last loop has broken, the end of the resectoscope sheath has become dangerously worn, or the diathermy machine has broken down. There must always be an adequate number of spares of the things that often go wrong, e.g. light leads, lamps, resectoscope loops and sheaths. Your hospital should always have several spare telescopes and at least one spare diathermy machine.

Telescopes

The story of the invention of the rod-lens telescope by the late Professor Harold Hopkins (Fig. 2.1), and of its development by Karl Storz, is now well known and has been told elsewhere[1]. What is not so well known is the reason why so many resectionists use a 30°

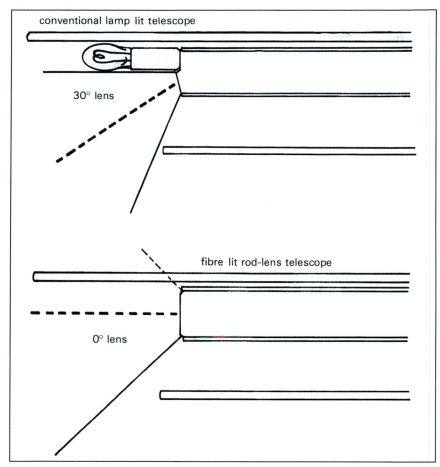

Figure 2.2
The filament lamp at the end of the telescope obliged one to use a 30° telescope.

rather than a forward-looking or 0° telescope (Fig. 2.2). Sixty years ago, because there was a tiny lamp at the end of the telescope, it was necessary to have a slightly angled line of vision: it was a matter of necessity, not choice. However it did make it slightly more easy to see the floor of the trough from which a chip of prostate had been taken. Newcomers to the art of transurethral resection will find it easier to use a 0° telescope from the beginning.

Sheaths

The early sheaths were made of bakelite, later of fibreglass and similar plastics which were apt to crack and split. Today sheaths are always made of steel, with an insulated tip made of plastic or ceramic (Fig. 2.3).

Figure 2.3
Steel sheath with ceramic tip.

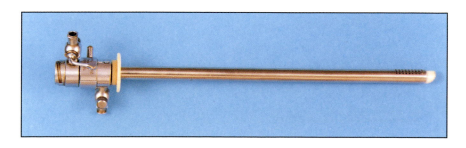

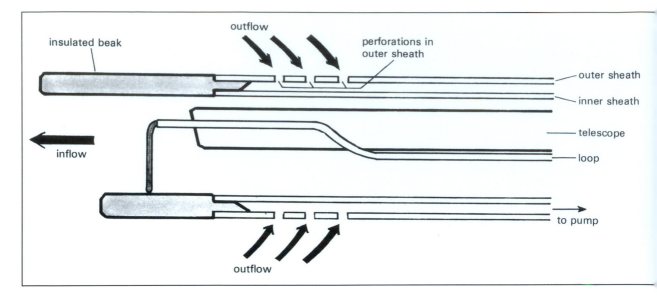

Figure 2.4
Iglesias's continuous irrigation.

Iglesias devised a continuous flow resectoscope[2] which allowed the irrigating fluid to be continually circulated in and out of the bladder to avoid build-up of pressure inside it, and to keep the field always clear (Fig. 2.4). A continuous flow resectoscope is particularly useful when resecting larger bladder tumours and to keep the field clear when demonstrating an operation.

Lighting

Modern flexible fibre-lighting is the result of another of Hopkins' inventions. Each glass fibre is coated with glass of a different refractive index, so that light entering at one end is totally internally reflected and emerges at the other. Repeated use of the cable results in fracture of the small glass fibres and gradually the cable transmits less light. Clumsy handling accelerates this process of wear and tear, but in time every cable must be replaced and there must always be spares.

Where the light lead is plugged into the source it becomes very hot and must be insulated to prevent staff handling the cable from getting burnt (Fig. 2.5). Absorption of the light at the other end of the cable by dark green drapes may result in local heating and even smouldering of the cloth which may give the patient a burn (Fig. 2.6), so that when not in use the end of the cable must always be kept well away from the patient.

It is equally important, when using some of the very bright light sources that are used for television, for the surgeon to safeguard his own retina: only the booby looks at the sun, and one must never allow the full intensity of the light reflected from the bladder to enter one's eye without interposing the teaching attachment or the beam splitter.

Figure 2.5
*Where the light cable joins
the light source it gets very
hot and must be insulated.*

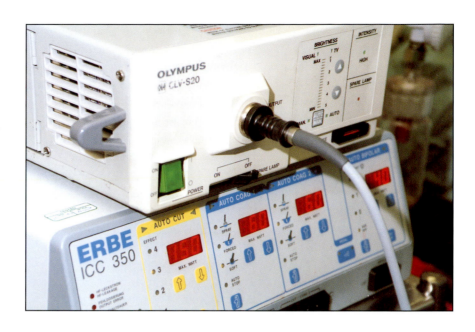

Figure 2.6
*If the light cable shines on
a dry sterile drape it can
smoulder and give the
patient a burn.*

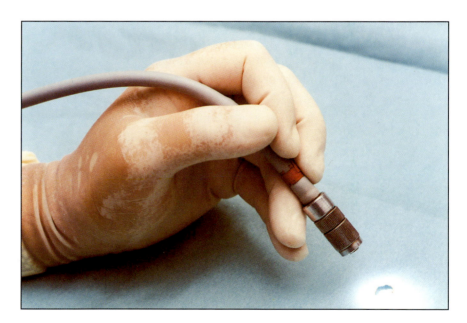

The handpiece

Nothing gives rise to more personal fads and fancies than the
particular design of the resectoscope handpiece. There are many to
choose from, and no one design is outstanding. What you need is a
handpiece that is strong, will stand up to wear and tear, and will go
on working smoothly in spite of much use. It is irritating and
sometimes dangerous when a handpiece sticks or jams in mid-cut.

Many surgeons today work with one finger in the rectum and there is an advantage in a spring action which returns the loop to the starting position without action on the part of the surgeon. There are also advantages in having all the cables on rotating attachments, so that the instrument can be rotated without obstructing or entangling the water pipes, light or diathermy cables.

Light sources

There are many different light sources on the market today. Curiously, they all come with a rheostat to allow the light input to be varied, even though everyone uses the maximum intensity the light can provide. Far more important than a rheostat is that there are plenty of spare lamps, and that everyone in the operating room team knows how to change them. Flash for endoscopic photography is useless.

Teaching equipment

Every surgeon is always a teacher, but to teach endoscopic surgery one must have the right equipment. Relatively cheap teaching attachments are available, made from a coordinated glass fibre cable or an articulated set of rod-lens telescopes, but both have been superseded today by a new generation of lightweight chip cameras which attach directly to the eyepiece of the telescope (Fig. 2.7) (see Chapter 3).

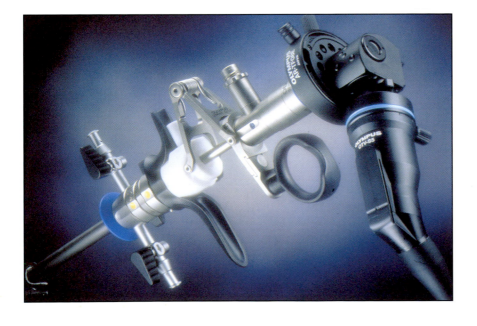

Figure 2.7
Modern chip camera with beam splitter. Courtesy of KeyMed (Olympus).

Diathermy

Transurethral resection requires a powerful diathermy machine which can both cut tissue and stop bleeding under water. If your budget is limited, economize on the resectoscope rather than the diathermy. Some of the diathermy machines which are adequate for haemostasis in general surgery will not cut under water.

Many of us take diathermy for granted: there is a big box with two pedals and some dials. When it does not work we ask the nurse to turn up the current. This is often exactly wrong, and diathermy is such an important part of the work of the urologist that he or she must understand its principles. The following account is intended to help the surgeon, even though it may occasionally offend the electrical engineer[3,4].

When an electric current passes between two contacts on the body there is always a certain increase in temperature in the tissues through which the current flows. This increase in temperature depends on the volume of tissue through which the current passes, the resistance of the tissues and the strength of the current. The stronger the current, the greater the rise in temperature.

When a direct current is switched on or off, nerves are stimulated and muscles will twitch. If the switching on and off is rapid enough, as with the Faradic current of a dynamo, there is the sustained contraction familiar to the physiology class as the 'tetanic contraction'.

If the frequency of the alternating current is increased beyond a certain critical level, there is no time for the cell membrane of nerve or muscle to become depolarized and nerves and muscles are no longer stimulated. The critical frequency depends to some extent on the strength of the current; with small currents it is of the order of 10 000 cycles per second (10 kHz). In practice much greater frequencies are used from 300 kHz to 5 MHz which today are generated by transistorized valve circuits.

With frequencies as great as this a very large current can be passed through the patient without exciting nerves or muscles, and it is then possible to exploit the heating effect at the points of contact. If one contact is made large, the heat is dissipated over a wide area and the rise of temperature is insignificant. Such a contact is the earth or neutral electrode under which the rise in temperature is only 1 or 2°C: it is the other end which concerns us, the working electrode or diathermy loop. This is kept deliberately thin so that the heating effect is maximum (Fig. 2.8).

The effect of the diathermy current on the tissues depends on the heat that is generated under the diathermy loop. The effect of heat on tissues is well known to us from everyday experience in the kitchen: when cooking an egg, at first the albumen turns white and shrivels as it coagulates. Then the egg fries, blackens and (in air) may smoke, crackle and eventually catch fire.

These changes are indeed seen in everyday open surgery, though even here it should be noted that good haemostasis depends on poaching, not roasting. It is the drying, coagulation and distortion of small blood vessels and plasma proteins which seals them. This requires only 'white coagulation'. Blackening and smoke are unnecessary and cause needless tissue necrosis.

If the current is increased to raise the temperature still further there is an explosive vaporization of intracellular water in the tissue. In transurethral resection this additional rise in temperature is

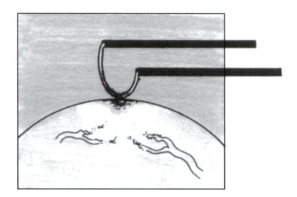

Figure 2.8
The coagulating current cooks the tissue for some distance around the loop and congeals the blood vessels.

achieved by a spark, the result of ionization of the water between the electrode and the tissue[3]. The electrode does not actually need to touch the tissue. The sparks explode the cells into steam, but their energy does not reach the deeper layers, so the cut is a clean one, but the blood vessels underneath are not sealed. The cutting current is a pure sine-wave current (Fig. 2.9).

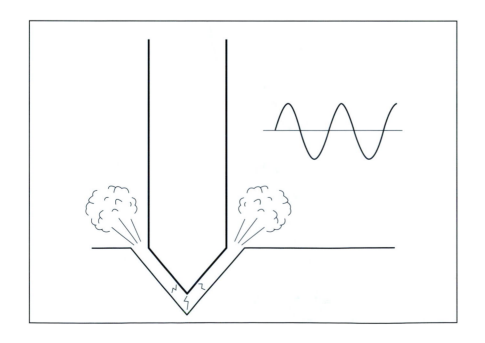

Figure 2.9
Cutting current: a continuous sine-wave.

Figure 2.10
Coagulating current; short bursts of sine-waves produce local heating and coagulation.

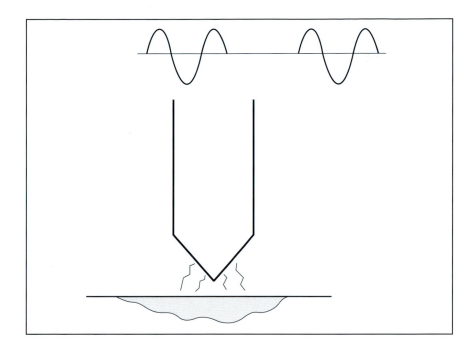

Coagulation is achieved in general with short bursts of sine waves which give longer sparks, but with intervals between them to allow the tissue to cool: the result is sustained heating which leads to poaching rather than explosion of the tissue (Fig. 2.10).

By designing the solid state generator to deliver a mixture of pure sine-wave 'cutting' and interrupted bursts of sine-wave currents for 'coagulation' a current can be designed to allow a combination of cutting and coagulation—the 'blended' current[3].

If a large electrode is used (as with the big roly-ball) there is a danger that the deeper layers of tissue will be cooked, since the heating effect is proportional to the square of the diameter of the contact. This must always be kept in mind when using the coagulating current in the vicinity of the sphincter (Fig. 2.11).

Figure 2.11
Too much coagulation with the roly-ball electrode can cause destruction of deeper tissues, e.g. the sphincter.

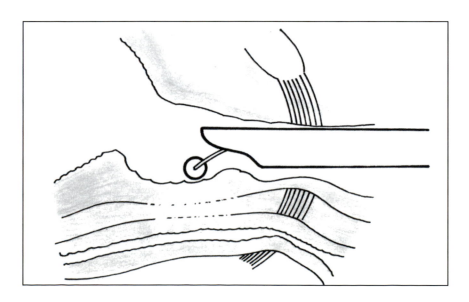

If the current does not seem to be stopping the bleeding, do not make the common mistake of asking for the current to be increased. The problem may be that it is sparking and causing explosion (cutting) of the underlying tissue. Turn it down.

Diathermy burns

If current returns to earth through a small contact rather than the broad area of the earth pad, then the tissues through which the current passes will be heated just like those under the cutting loop. If the pad is making good contact, the current will find it easier to run to earth through the pad and no harm will arise even when there is accidental contact with some metal object.

The real danger arises when the diathermy pad is not making good contact with the patient. It may not be plugged in, its wire may be broken (Fig. 2.12) or, in the older type of earth plate, the conductive jelly may have dried out. Under these circumstances the current must find its way to earth somehow, and any contact may then become the site of a dangerous rise in temperature.

It follows that if the diathermy does not seem to be working, the first thing that the surgeon must *not* do is to ask for an increase in current. Instead, check that the diathermy plate is making good contact with the skin of the patient; check that the lead is undamaged; check that the resectoscope loop is securely fixed to the contact (Fig. 2.13). Many modern diathermy machines have a warning circuit which sounds an alarm when there is imperfect contact between the earth plate and the patient (Fig. 2.14): others have a very low capacitance between the diathermy machine and earth, so that if the earth plate is not attached the current finds it easier to run to earth than through the patient: the surgeon finds the loop does not cut, but the patient cannot be burnt.

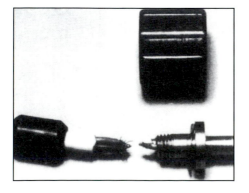

Figure 2.12
The wire may be frayed inside its insulation; always check the circuit from pad to diathermy machine if the loop does not cut.

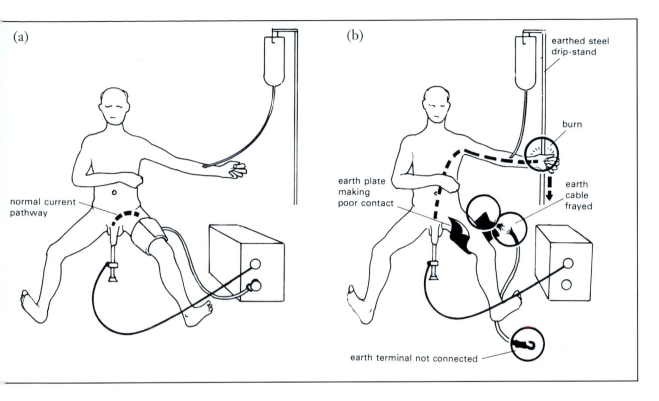

Figure 2.13
(a) Normal current pathway from loop to earth plate.
(b) If the earth circuit is interrupted, current will find its way via any accidental small metal contact and cause a burn.

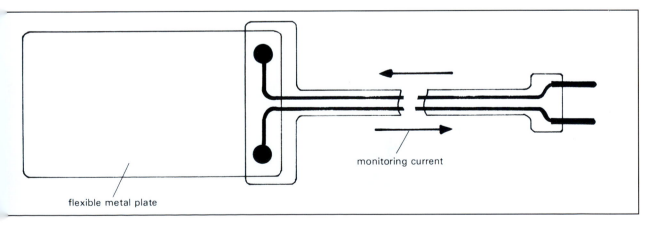

Figure 2.14
Safety circuit incorporated in dry plate; if the circuit is interrupted there is a warning signal, but this does not mean that the plate has been applied to the patient.

Pacemakers

An increasing number of elderly men come up for prostatectomy with pacemakers (Fig. 2.15). Four types are in common use[5,6]:

1. Fixed-rate pacemakers for patients with permanent heart block: these stimulate the ventricle at a constant rate.

2. Demand pacemakers, which detect ventricular contraction, amplify it, and feed it back to the ventricle. Only if the ventricular impulse is too weak to be detected will the pacemaker deliver its own regular beat.

3. Atrial synchronous pacemakers have one electrode in the atrium which detects a contraction arising there, and a second electrode in the ventricle to supply it with the amplified impulse. If the atrial contractions become too frequent a fixed-rate system takes over.

4. Atrioventricular sequential pacemakers stimulate the atria at a variable but appropriate rate.

The earlier demand pacemakers could sometimes be deceived by the diathermy current into delivering a rate of stimulation that was dangerously high. The modern devices can instead be inhibited by the high frequency diathermy current, so that the patient may get no pacing at all while the diathermy is activated.

The precautions are not difficult: the patient plate should be sited so that the current path does not go right through the pacemaker.

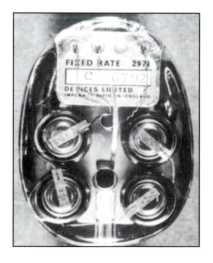

Figure 2.15
Cardiac pacemaker.

The diathermy machine should be placed well away from the pacemaker. The heartbeat should be continually monitored, and a defibrillator and external pacemaker should be at hand. Experience over many years of performing transurethral resection on men with pacemakers has led to the following routine: (Fig. 2.16)

1. Consult with the cardiologist to verify the type of pacemaker in use.
2. Have an ECG running throughout the operation.
3. Make sure a defibrillator and external pacemaker are available.
4. Give systemic antibiotics to avoid bacterial colonization of the pacemaker during the TUR.
5. Because the pacemaker-driven heart will not respond to fluid overload in the normal way, the resection should be as quick as possible, and fluid overload should be avoided (Fig. 2.17).

Figure 2.16
Hazards to be avoided when using diathermy in a patient with a pacemaker.

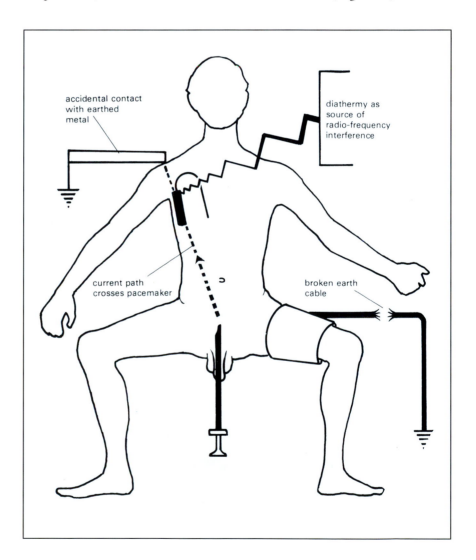

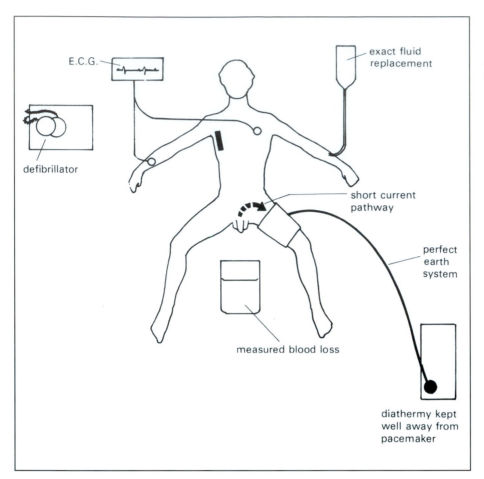

Figure 2.17
Precautions to take when performing TUR in a man with a pacemaker.

Labels in figure:
- E.C.G.
- exact fluid replacement
- defibrillator
- short current pathway
- perfect earth system
- measured blood loss
- diathermy kept well away from pacemaker

Sterilization

The instruments used in urological surgery should, in theory, be no less sterile than those used to operate on the eye or the brain. There is only one way to guarantee the destruction of all known microorganisms, and that is by heat. The ideal method would be to put all the instruments through an oven or an autoclave as is the normal practice for haemostatic forceps and retractors. There are also many parts of the ordinary urological armamentarium, e.g. the metal cystoscope and resectoscope sheath, the taps, obturators, etc., which could and should ideally be sterilized by heat, but in practice the autoclave cycle is slow, and few urological departments could afford enough instruments to run a busy list of endoscopic operations if they all had to be autoclaved between cases.

Again, many instruments are exceptionally delicate and costly. Telescopes are a particular example: if subjected to heat, the expansion of the metal sheath and the glass lenses being different, they work loose. Repairs are costly because the instrument has virtually to be rebuilt from scratch.

Francis[7] devised a 'pasteurizer' which heated the instruments to 70°C for 10 min. He proved that this would kill off vegetative organisms and most viruses, but not spores. Since spore-born infection is almost unknown in the urinary tract, the Francis Pasteurizer offered a useful compromise and many rod-lens telescopes are now available which will withstand pasteurization.

There have been many attempts to use vapour for sterilization. Adding formalin vapour to low pressure steam at 80°C was found to kill spores as well as vegetative organisms[8] but the necessary equipment failed so often that the method fell into disrepute.

Ethylene oxide gas at 80°C was equally effective, but needed expensive plant and the dangers of explosion and toxicity precluded it for use between cases[9].

Inevitably urologists have turned to some form of chemical sterilization, but always come up against the well known problem of Fleming's 'artificial wound', i.e. the crevices between screws and hinges where bacteria can lurk out of the reach of any kind of antiseptic solution.

At present activated glutaraldehyde is widely used. For it to reach microorganisms every screw and tap must be taken apart, and care must be taken that the liquid is forced through every channel. Contact may give rise to severe dermatitis, and inhalation may cause respiratory illness in staff. Better means of chemical sterilization are being actively sought, but the target has yet to be reached[10]. Various manufacturers now market autoclavable telescopes but their life span is not yet clearly determined.

References

1. Blandy JP, Fowler CG. Lower tract endoscopy. *Br Med Bull* 1986; **42**: 280.
2. Iglesias JJ, Stams UK. How to prevent the TUR syndrome. *Urologe* 1975; **14**: 287.
3. Fowler CG. Urological technology. In: Blandy JP, Fowler CG *Urology*. 2nd edn. Oxford: Blackwell Science, 1996; 3–17.
4. Mitchell JP, Lumb GN. *A Handbook of Surgical Diathermy*. Bristol: Wright, 1966.
5. Sowton E. Use of cardiac pacemakers in Britain. *Br Med J* 1976; **2**: 1182.
6. Spurrell RAJ. Cardiac pacemakers. *Br J Clin Equipment* 1975; **1**: 43.
7. Francis AE. The use of a pasteurising water bath for disinfection of cystoscopes. *J Urol* 1961; **86**: 679.
8. Alder VG, Brown AM, Gillespie WA. Disinfection of heat sensitive material by low temperature steam and formaldehyde. *J Clin Path* 1966; **19**: 83.
9. Kelsey JC. Sterilisation by ethylene oxide. *J Clin Path* 1961; **14**: 59.
10. Cooke RPD, Feneley RCL, Ayliffe G *et al.* Decontamination of urological equipment: interim report of a working group of the Standing Committee on Urological Instruments of BAUS. *Br J Urol* 1993; **71**: 5.

Chapter 3
Closed circuit television for the urologist

Closed circuit colour television (CCTV) is now widely used by urologists in the United Kingdom. Few urological surgeons now crane their necks to put an eye to the telescope of their instruments, preferring to sit comfortably looking at the colour monitor conveniently placed in front of them (Fig. 3.1). They thus protect their cervical discs[1] and lessen the risk of facial contamination by blood and irrigant[2].

Urological trainees receive formal training in monitored transurethral resection as courses are run regularly around the country using CCTV for endoscopy. The improved technology of the miniature chip camera provides such an excellent image that it is now possible to see on the TV screen as much detail—perhaps even more—than one can see by looking directly into the telescope of the instrument. Not only transurethral resection can be done as a 'monitored' procedure, but all varieties of urological endoscopy, urethroscopy, cystoscopy, ureteroscopy and pyeloscopy are probably done more easily and effectively using the CCTV camera and working from the monitor.

The urologist who wishes to set up CCTV for use in the operating theatre is faced by a bewildering choice of television equipment. Many manufacturers provide comprehensive packages and it is difficult to choose between them on any grounds other than cost. Ask yourself six basic questions:

1. What do you think you want?
2. What do you think you need?

Figure 3.1
(a) One monitor is placed over the patient.
(b) The second monitor is on the wall.

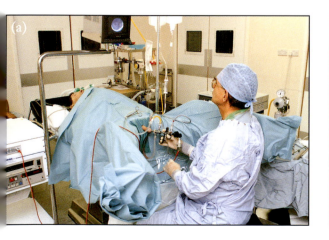

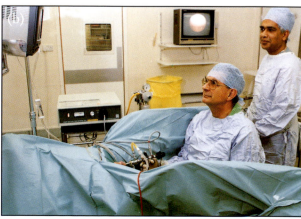

3. Where will you get it from?
4. Should you buy a package?
5. How much will it cost?
6. What will it cost to run?

What do you think you want?

It is clear that a CCTV set up in the operating theatre is worthwhile. Apart from saving your neck and helping to protect you from infection by hepatitis and HIV viruses by lessening the risk of facial contamination, CCTV enables you to teach trainees and demonstrate endoscopic technique to theatre personnel. But which parts of the rather expensive system are vital and which are luxuries? You must decide what you want to achieve. The basic wish is to project an image of what the telescope sees onto a TV screen. This may be for a number of reasons. Staff who work in an operating room where almost all the operations are invisible to anyone but the surgeon find it boring. Being able to see what is going on kindles interest. They can see which instrument is going to be needed next and thus anticipate your wishes. There may be students or junior staff to teach. Perhaps you would like to make videotapes for teaching or demonstration purposes[3]. Above all, you may simply want to protect your health. All these are valid reasons to consider the installation of CCTV in the urology operating theatre, but it can be difficult to differentiate between need and luxury.

What do urologists need?

To use CCTV in an operating theatre you need:
1. The usual endoscopic and diathermy equipment.
2. A light source with sufficient output to permit the use of a TV camera; a dim light provides a poor TV image. Your eye can accommodate a dim light because it is an infinitely more efficient optical instrument than the camera.
3. Fibroptic cables capable of conducting the higher intensity illumination from the light source to the endoscope without suffering heat damage.
4. A good quality telescope. All telescopes deteriorate with use; endoscopic TV needs a really clear telescope. A hazy telescope gives a poor TV image, even if your eye copes adequately.
5. A TV camera.
6. A video monitor or monitors.
7. Some form of constant irrigation system. It is perfectly possible to use CCTV with intermittent irrigation, but constant irrigation enables the watcher to see an uninterrupted operation.

8. Some sort of trolley or cabinet to contain the camera and its ancillary works. This is not essential, but video equipment is expensive and relatively fragile and a trolley is a good way of protecting your investment. The above list does not include any recording equipment; recording the TV image is not a necessity. It is something to which most urological surgeons will come, but not until they have mastered the general technique of CCTV for endoscopic surgery and have decided what they wish to record and why. This will be discussed later.

Light sources

A suitable general purpose high output light source, either high intensity tungsten, metal halide or xenon arc, can be purchased from the urological instrument dealer without difficulty. Tungsten light sources put out between 50 and 150 watts and suit many modern chip TV cameras, but are at the lower end of the spectrum of suitability for CCTV and may not give the best images under adverse operating conditions. Metal halide sources usually operate at 250 watts and xenon arc sources at over 300 watts. Any of these can be used as the standard endoscopic illumination, whether the TV is being used or not, so it is not necessary to have a conventional light source as well. However, a word of caution; high powered light sources produce light of such intensity that the heat produced can burn holes in surgical drapes, or in patients, if the cable is left unattended (Fig. 3.2).

Figure 3.2
Make sure the light cable does not come in contact with the drape.

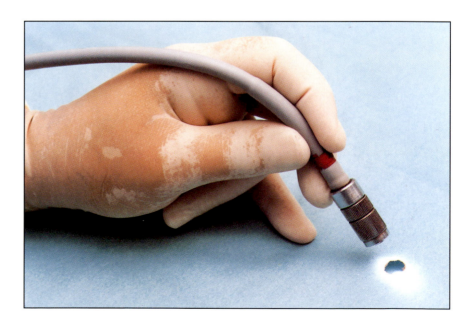

The lamps are expensive and benefit from a little thought and care; do not turn them off at the end of each operation, as maximum wear on the light source occurs each time it is activated. Lamps will last longer if they are turned on at the start of the list and left on until the last case is finished. Always keep a spare lamp and ensure that you know how to change it so that the teaching session does not come to an untimely halt due to a burned out lamp.

As an alternative to a general purpose light source, it is possible to buy a 'dedicated' light source designed to work with a specific TV camera; these come as part of various CCTV 'packages'. The advantage of these dedicated metal halide or xenon arc sources is that they are linked electronically with the camera to produce an image of standard brightness. Feed back from camera to light source gives more light when the field is dark and reduces the light to prevent highlight and flare when the subject matter is over-illuminated. It is a more expensive option than a general purpose light source and it has been the authors' experience that general purpose light sources work well enough, especially if minimizing the capital outlay is important.

Light cables

Armoured, specially insulated, or fluid–filled light cables are widely available. They work just as well with low light intensities, so if CCTV is going to be used one might as well standardize all the cables to be capable of carrying high intensity light, particularly if you plan to use only a high intensity light source. Ensure that the cables are in good condition for TV work; broken fibres and the inevitable melt damage which occurs at the source terminal of the cable are important causes of a poor TV image.

Telescopes

It goes without saying that only rod lens telescopes are suitable for TV work. The slow deterioration of a rod lens telescope from normal regular use is imperceptible to the eye until it is very advanced as the eye is an altogether superior optical instrument to any TV camera. By the time a telescope looks dim to the eye, it is probably incapable of transmitting an image which the TV camera can visualize at all. You must use a telescope in 'new' condition if CCTV is to be used.

Trolleys

It is essential to house the delicate CCTV equipment safely. This can be in the wall of the operating room, with long cables to the camera, or it can be in a mobile trolley or cabinet, perhaps with an extensible arm to support the 'resecting' monitor (Fig. 3.3). The less it is necessary to manhandle the equipment the less the risk of accidental damage. It is advisable to be able to lock the equipment into its housing, not only to prevent theft, but also to reduce the incidence of malfunction due to knob-twiddling by TV 'experts' or by accidental alteration of switches.

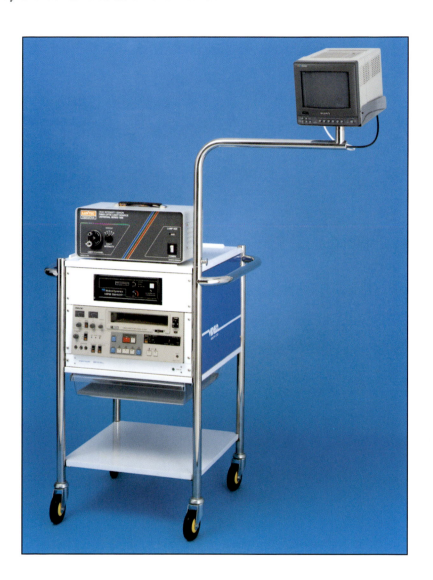

Figure 3.3
Purpose-built cabinet with arm to support monitor. Courtesy of Video South Medical TV.

Constant irrigation systems

Constant irrigation with continuous removal of the irrigant during prostatic or bladder tumour resection keeps the TV image constant and makes it easier for an observer to follow. This can be achieved by an irrigating resectoscope sheath (the authors' preference) or a suprapubic cannula system. Intermittent irrigation means that the teaching process has to be interrupted every time the bladder fills and has to be emptied, making the teaching less effective and the operation slower because the surgeon has to find his place again after emptying of the bladder.

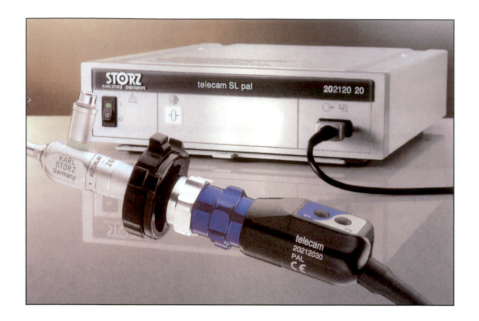

Figure 3.4
*A direct coupled camera.
Courtesy of K. Storz.*

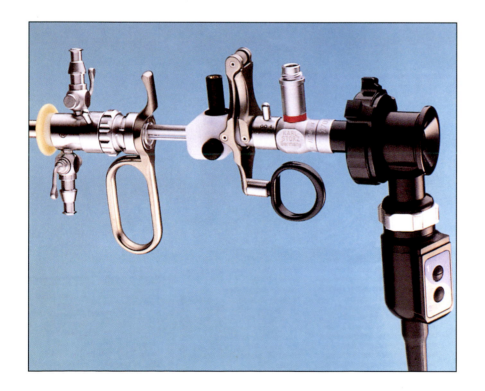

Figure 3.5
*A fitted beam splitter
keeps the camera steady
and the image the right
way up. Courtesy of K.
Storz.*

Cameras

A modern three-element (each element now being a chip, formerly a tube) television camera produces the best image with regard to colour, crispness and resolution, but it is a bulky piece of equipment which does not lend itself to use in an urological operating room without a squad of assistants, cannot be coupled directly to the endoscope because of its size and has to be used through a jointed beam splitter. There is inevitable rotation at the joints with consequent loss of orientation of the TV image.

Modern single-chip cameras are small enough to fit directly onto the endoscope eyepiece without making it too clumsy to manipulate. They produce a remarkably clear image, with excellent depth of focus and colour reproduction. They can also be made waterproof, to allow disinfection by soaking. If the surgeon wants to operate by direct vision, using a beam splitter, this is not jointed and the problems of image orientation are minimal.

Basically only four chips are commercially available for chip cameras, so whatever camera one buys it will have one of them. They all have very similar performance. What else one gets will depend on what the manufacturer has decided to provide. A hand-held camera purchased in the High Street shop has all its working parts in one box—so it is relatively bulky—much too big for the urologist's purposes. In an endoscopic camera the chip has been separated from the works and connected by a cable.

Some camera manufacturers use a 12 volt system to power the camera for reasons of safety. Some put in zoom fitments. Some include colour bar generators. Some have automatic light balance. However, the signal processing is going to be what the chip manufacturer supplies so that, on the whole, modern chip cameras have fairly comparable performance and the urologist must look for what he wants.

Cameras may be made to couple directly onto the telescope eyepiece (Fig. 3.4), or may be attached via a right-angled beam splitter (Fig. 3.5). A direct coupled camera will rotate with the telescope so that the image will rotate on the monitor. To keep it still the camera must be held steady and not rotated with the endoscope; this needs an extra hand. As most urological surgeons like to use both hands on the endoscope this is inconvenient. A fitted beam splitter is more convenient as it will either swing on the eyepiece or have an inbuilt rotation point that keeps the camera steady in relation to the telescope, so that the image is always kept the right way up.

Monitors

Video monitors come in all sizes and qualities. As a general principle, the picture will be clearer and sharper if a monitor is purchased rather than a television set. So, if the salesman tells you that the 'monitor' can be used as a television set, you know you will not get the highest quality picture, however convenient it may be to watch the tennis when things get tedious. The size and number of monitors provided in the operating room is a personal (and financial) choice. It is the authors' experience that it is unwise to have a wall monitor with less than a 28 inch screen, and that two monitors, facing in opposite directions, are better than one. A 10 to 14 inch monitor is large enough to resect with, and can be easily suspended above the patient's abdomen for ease of use (Fig. 3.1). It is best to have this small 'resecting' monitor working on 12 volts in case it gets wet, to minimize the risk of electrocution of patient or surgeon.

Recording equipment

Recording equipment can provide videotape or still pictures. It comes in all the packages on offer. The video recorders can provide the U-matic format, VHS or 8 mm. Expensive or less expensive still picture printers are available; cost being directly related to performance. You should think carefully before spending your money and ask whether you really need any of these facilities. What do you want to record? What will you do with the recordings when you have made them?

If a recording is needed for the records then a still printer is required—for something like a bladder tumour, for instance. But it is difficult to show the whole of a bladder tumour on one print if it is more than 1 cm across. It is necessary to take a long view of a sizeable tumour to keep it in frame. The human eye can cope with the inverse square law, being a better optical instrument, but the video camera cannot, and a large object cannot be illuminated adequately to produce a video image suitable for printing. The still video printer is an expensive luxury and only one of the new digital recorders will provide prints that are good enough for publication (as in this book) but are mightily expensive as well as being prodigal of computer space.

If the requirement is to keep a tape for a medico–legal record, the tape must be complete and unexpurgated. It will therefore be long (and boring to watch) and a consideration will be the cost of the videotape and the problem of storage. Videotape intended for lectures or teaching requires some method of editing the tape so that it is concise and interesting. That means at least another video cassette recorder, and it is not possible to get a tidily edited tape simply by cross-recording from one tape to another by using two

VCRs. To edit a videotape properly requires an editing suite in which a computer links and controls the two VCRs. Videotape editing involves re-recording the scenes to be kept, in the order that is required, on a second tape (unlike ciné film editing when the film is physically cut with scissors and rejoined). Without computerized coordination of the two VCRs the end result is uneven and the joins between the re-recorded scenes are obtrusive. Such an editing suite is expensive, but you must have access to one because you must do the editing yourself, or supervise it personally, to achieve the result you require.

The urologist setting up CCTV in the operating room should postpone the purchase of recording equipment until the system is installed and running. You may never want to record. Prints are of no great value. Making a videotape is time consuming: it takes at least an hour and a half of editing and sound recording time to create 15 minutes of final tape, in addition to the time spent making the original video recording. It is also very expensive.

If you have decided to purchase a video cassette recorder and make videotapes the next step is to decide on the recording format. At present (1998) three formats are available: U-matic (both low and high band), VHS (and now Super-VHS) and Video 8 (and High 8). U-matic provides the best colour and picture detail; the tape moves relatively slowly and the amount of electronic information stored on each 'frame' is considerable, but the VCRs and tapes are bulky and expensive and the longest is only 1 hour in length. High band U-matic equipment is not entirely compatible with low band equipment, which is now not manufactured.

VHS machines and tapes are cheaper and less bulky and the tapes are much longer, but the colour and detail were noticeably inferior to U-matic until the introduction of Super-VHS, which is now nearer to U-matic quality. Eight millimetre video, Video 8 and High 8, are less satisfactory and not available for endoscopic use in any case. Video formats come and go, with constant development and improvement. The best advice is to try what is available locally, see what each format offers and make a decision to suit your own needs. Do not forget that TV standards vary from country to country and from continent to continent. In the United Kingdom the standard is PAL, in Europe it is mainly SECAM; both of these are similar in quality, but not compatible. In the Americas the standard is NTSC, which gives an inferior picture quality, both in detail and colour, and is compatible with neither PAL nor SECAM. Videotapes made in the United States of America cannot therefore be screened in England, and vice versa, without conversion, which is expensive and reduces the quality of the final tape.

When video-recording is required, for whatever reason, make sure your camera has a colour bar generator. An unused videotape—the tape which looks like a snowstorm if it is played—has no electronic information on it. The computer which matches the speed of the tapes and the pictures during the editing process needs some reference point on the accepting tape. 'Snowstorm' tape does not have such a reference point on it, so the computer has to guess, and may guess wrong. By recording colour bars for the whole length of each new tape a square wave, the control track, is added along the tape to which the editing computer can refer, permitting a cleanly edited end result. So, if making videotapes is the aim, which will by definition need editing, life is made easier if the camera has a colour bar generator.

Of course, once the decision is made to start making videotapes one is risking a serious addiction. It is a habit which costs endless money, fills the office with equipment and wastes hours of spare time. However, it can be very rewarding and it is undoubtedly a marvellous teaching method. Videotapes can be used again and again, so that when the procedure being taught has been overtaken by the inevitable progress of surgery the tape can be re-used, unlike ciné-film. Video is an instant medium—the results are immediately available and can be re-recorded if the scene is not exactly what is required, unlike ciné-film which has to be developed before the recording can be seen. Videotape tends to deteriorate if stored without being played from time to time as the electronic information stored upon it tends to 'leach' onto the contiguous tape on the reel. Archived tape therefore needs regular attention.

Where do urologists buy their CCTV equipment?

It is possible to purchase remarkably inexpensive closed circuit colour television equipment from the shops in the High Street. Good VHS and Video 8 cameras and editing equipment are available in a wide choice, and excellent bargains can be found by shopping around if the requirements are known. If all that you need is a system which will show scenes in theatre and open operations then the High Street shops can provide everything. It is possible to set up a ward or classroom teaching module relatively inexpensively in this way. Single chip soakable cameras cannot be bought in the High Street, nor can U-matic format recording equipment. For these, the urologist must go to one of the specialist firms[4].

The best advice for the urologist seeking to put a CCTV system into the operating theatre is to try out all the equipment that is available from all the firms who sell it. See how each performs in your hands in your own operating room; decide what suits your requirements, and purchase as your budget permits. Since the cost of individual items of equipment are comparable wherever they are purchased it is more important to find out which firm will offer service and repair arrangements; find out if the equipment has to go to Alaska for repair, or if it can be done locally, because one may take longer than the other. And wherever it does go, will the firm provide a loan replacement part to keep the CCTV system in action?

Should the urologist buy a CCTV package?

CCTV for the urological surgeon is provided by specialist suppliers. Most of these suppliers will provide a package which usually consists of their camera and beam splitter, a light source (which may or may not be dedicated) and a VCR. In many cases the package is enclosed in a trolley or cabinet of the supplier's own design, often of a modular pattern which can be varied to accommodate special requirements.

Most suppliers are open to negotiation as to the exact contents of their package. Most offer alternative format VCRs, or will leave it out of the package altogether. Some offer still image recorders. Most will agree to exclude the light source if the surgeon already has a suitable one, although the dedicated light source suppliers make the point that their camera works best with its own dedicated light source.

There are suppliers who will come to see what is required and are then prepared to put together a package to suit your requirements, subject to including their camera in the package. For this it is necessary for you to know what you want and to have had some experience in the use of CCTV, which might perhaps be called 'second generation' CCTV usage. Of course, if you do have experience in the use of CCTV and know all about electronics, go shopping for the necessary components and put together your own package and so save money. However, few surgeons have such expertise and you will find that the suppliers offer a good deal with good performance from most of their packages. The vital thing is to have an extended trial of the package on offer before purchase—if the supplier will not agree to this then go elsewhere.

How much does it all cost?

The cost of CCTV for urology will depend on where you work and whether the equipment is made locally or has to be imported. The most expensive equipment is not necessarily the best for your particular purpose. Look at the equipment that is available in your area; make sure that it is really what you want; compare the costs and try each set of equipment out. Discover the servicing arrangements on offer. You will then be in the best position to purchase a system which works for you and is within your budget.

What are the costs of running a CCTV system?

It is important to have a clear idea what it will cost to run a CCTV system in the urology operating room or department. Once purchased and installed, electronic equipment is not expensive to run. The consumption of electricity is minimal. Some parts of the system have batteries which need to be replaced from time to time at nominal cost. If recording is to be done the cost of tapes must be added. Apart from these considerations there are no significant revenue implications of running a CCTV system, which is important information for the purchaser, whether this be the urology department, the Supplies Officer of the hospital or a Charity providing the equipment. If good equipment is purchased and reasonable care is taken of it, it will cost no more to run than a domestic TV or Hi Fi system.

It is essential to plan ahead in order to replace your equipment as time goes by because it will wear out and occasional unexpected breakdowns will occur. So keep spares where possible, particularly a light source lamp, and maintain a reserve of cash so that it is possible to replace parts rapidly and so keep the set-up going. Buy your equipment from someone who will offer a prompt and reliable repair and replacement service: you may wish to take out a service contract, but watch the price and be prepared to bargain.

Equipment with knobs attracts fiddlers like flies to rotten meat, and manufacturers seem impelled to fit multiple knobs on the front of all TV equipment for sales reasons. This lures the fiddler, who is usually a self-professed expert on all matters televisual. When the knob-fiddler has maladjusted everything in sight it can appear that the system has broken down. If the supplier is then called in to rescue the situation it can be expensive for what is actually simple adjustment. So wage war on fiddlers: fit locks, close doors, put up notices and, most important of all, learn how to do the adjustments. Anything which can be locked away after being set up and is thus invisible is an advantage.

Enthusiastic dusters are also a potential problem, changing the setting of a switch, perhaps from PAL to SECAM, at the flick of a wrist. Dust covers and lids help, but take care not to operate electronic equipment under its plastic cover because it may overheat and malfunction. Likewise do not keep electronic equipment in a cold place and expect it to work instantly in a warm room, condensation being a potent cause of malfunction.

Diathermy and other interference

Diathermy interference is a mysterious and troublesome pheno-menon which has plagued every urologist who has tried to set up CCTV in the operating theatre. Diathermy machines produce radio frequency waves which get transmitted around the theatre, the various leads being excellent aerials. Operating rooms have wiring systems producing electrical fields capable of generating interference on CCTV systems, as may electrical equipment in an adjoining room. A surgeon hoping to use CCTV must try out the system in his own operating room. If the interference cannot be eliminated easily, do not buy that system. If interference appears when it was not there before, check that all electrical connections are clean and firm, that no lead is frayed or its insulating cover damaged, and that the various pieces of equipment are properly earthed; this check should be applied to all the electrical equipment in the operating room, and especially to the diathermy. If interference persists after an extensive check of all leads, etc., get the diathermy checked electrically as it may be that a minor circuit malfunction has developed.

References

1. Whitaker RH, Green NA, Notley RG. Is cervical spondylosis an occupational hazard for urologists? *Brit J Urol*. 1983; **55**: 585–8.
2. McNicholas TA, Jones DJ, Sibley GN. AIDS: the contamination risk in urological surgery. *Brit J Urol*. 1989; **63**: 565–8.
3. O'Boyle PJ. Video-endoscopy: the remote operating technique. *Brit J Urol*. 1990; **65**: 557–9.
4. O'Boyle PJ, Raina S, Holdoway AT. Videoprostatectomy: guidelines for choosing an effective microvideo operating system. *Brit J Urol*. 1989; **63**: 624–6.

Chapter 4
Indications and preparations for transurethral resection

Transurethral resection is today the standard technique for the treatment of more than 90% of men with outflow obstruction of the bladder, whether it is caused by benign enlargement of the prostate, bladder neck dyssynergia or carcinoma. In addition, some 80% of cases of bladder cancer, where the tumour is superficial and well-differentiated, can and should be managed endoscopically. The preparations and precautions which are needed in all these cases are very similar. In this chapter we will be considering the routine preparations for transurethral resection for benign enlargement of the prostate.

Benign enlargement of the prostate

The prostate gland is made of two parts, an inner cranial zone and an outer caudal zone[1] (Fig. 4.1). Benign enlargement begins in the inner cranial zone in the collection of glands adjacent to the urethra[2]. No man can escape the changes which begin to occur in his prostate as he grows older: by the time he is 40 years old the microscope will show scores of tiny benign foci of nodular hyperplasia scattered throughout the inner zone of the gland.

Figure 4.1
The prostate has two zones; the inner mainly gives rise to benign hyperplasia, the outer (mainly) to carcinoma.

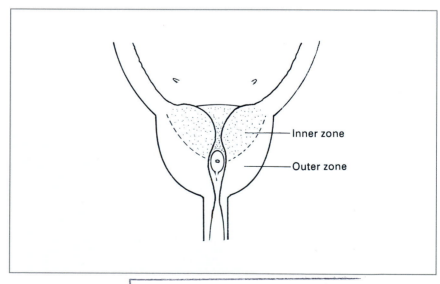

Inner zone

Outer zone

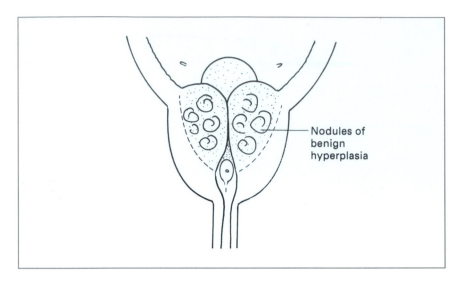

Figure 4.2
Nodules of hyperplasia begin to form in the inner zone, displacing the outer zone into the so-called 'surgical capsule'.

Nodules of benign hyperplasia

Over the next 30 years these foci gradually enlarge, coalesce and elongate the prostate, whilst compressing the prostatic urethra from side to side (Fig. 4.2). The enlargement of these nodules gives rise to the so-called lobes of the prostate, which are not a normal anatomical entity, but an artefact which reflects the way the bladder neck and the shape of the bony pelvis mould the enlarging adenoma. Transurethral resection aims to remove the enlarged inner zone tissue, leaving the outer zone more or less intact[3].

There is an equally important change in the smooth muscle at the neck of the bladder (Fig. 4.3), which loses its normal ability to relax in coordination with the contraction of the detrusor. The result is an

(a)   (b)

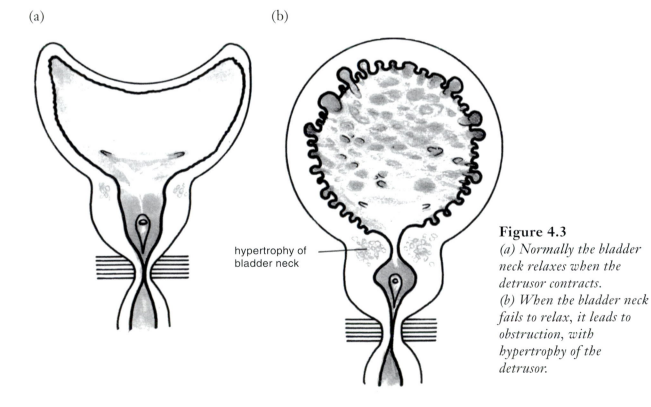

hypertrophy of bladder neck

Figure 4.3
(a) Normally the bladder neck relaxes when the detrusor contracts.
(b) When the bladder neck fails to relax, it leads to obstruction, with hypertrophy of the detrusor.

unyielding ring of tissue at the neck of the bladder which fails to open as the detrusor contracts. The combination of mechanical deformity and smooth muscle malfunction results in an increased resistance at the outlet of the bladder[4].

In response to this, the detrusor muscle undergoes hypertrophy (Fig. 4.4). To the naked eye the changes are obvious: the muscle thickens, and its trabeculae become coarsened and change from a fine feltwork into a net through whose spaces the mucosa of the bladder is pushed out to form multiple saccules and eventually diverticula.

Under the microscope there are more subtle changes: collagen is laid down between the smooth muscle fibres of the detrusor, and the connections between one muscle cell and its neighbours become altered[5]. In time, the detrusor begins to fail. Failure may be gradual or sudden. In gradual failure, at first the bladder is no longer capable of ridding itself of urine, with the tell-tale appearance in the ultrasound and urogram of residual urine (Fig. 4.5). This process may continue slowly and painlessly until one day the volume of residual urine becomes so great that the bladder begins to leak involuntarily—chronic retention with overflow.

In acute failure of the detrusor the patient suddenly finds himself unable to empty the bladder. This may occur at any stage in the story, and may be precipitated by some other illness, overdistension of the bladder from drunkenness or being given a diuretic.

Figure 4.4

(a) Saccules form when the urothelium bulges out between the hypertrophied trabeculae of detrusor. (b) Large saccules that bulge outside the detrusor form diverticula.

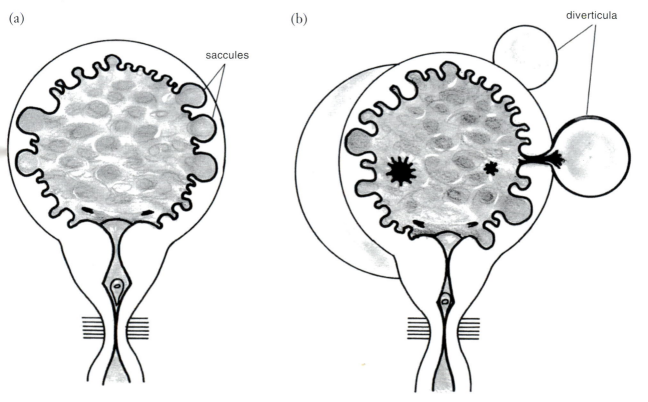

(a)   (b)

saccules

diverticula

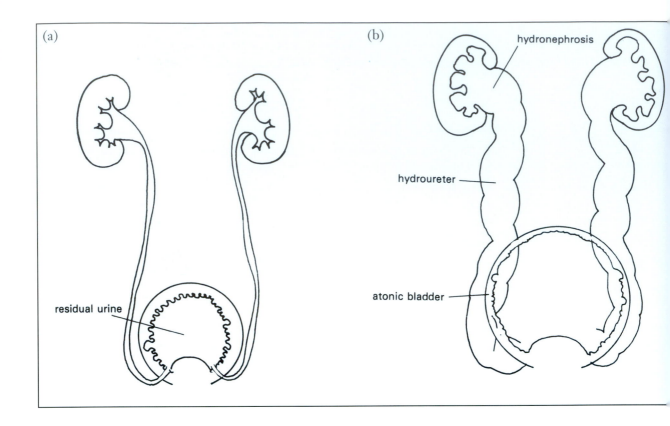

Quite early on in the progress of prostatic outflow obstruction, the increase in voiding pressure in the bladder may cause functional obstruction to the ureters, although it may be difficult to detect[4]. Later on as the full blown picture of chronic retention unfolds, the trigone is distorted by the enlarging adenoma, lifting up and obstructing the lower ends of the ureters. Hydroureter is succeeded by hydronephrosis, one side often becoming dilated before the other (Fig. 4.6). With hydronephrosis there is progressive flattening of the renal papillae and loss of the ability of the tubules to concentrate or acidify the urine. Step by step the patient is led to the stage where he is unable to concentrate his urine and develops an obligatory diuresis. His thirst mechanism may be impaired, so that when he arrives in hospital he may be seriously dehydrated.

If not corrected, the progressive back-pressure leads to impairment of glomerular filtration and at last there is a measurable elevation of blood urea and creatinine.

The indications for prostatectomy become more and more pressing as the progress of obstruction is continued. In the earliest stages, when the only effect of a slight increase in outflow resistance is a little hypertrophy of the detrusor, which may lead to uninhibited detrusor contractions (*detrusor instability*), the patient's only

Figure 4.5
Progressive deterioration of the detrusor:
(a) the muscle is hypertrophied, with trabeculation and saccules but only a small volume of residual urine.
(b) As the detrusor fails, there is a large volume of residual urine and obstructed ureters.

Figure 4.6
Typical IVU in advanced prostatic obstruction with large residual urine and bilateral hydronephrosis.

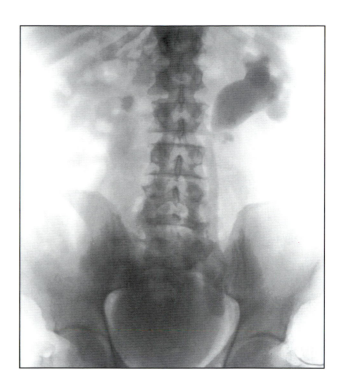

complaint is of some increased frequency and urgency of micturition. There is some evidence that relief of obstruction at this early stage may give better symptomatic results but one should be exceedingly cautious before offering the patient any operation, merely because of the symptom of frequency, unless there is clear urodynamic evidence of outflow obstruction (see page 52).

In a previous generation the prevailing mortality for any form of prostatectomy was so high that it was easy to show that certain episodes in the natural history of prostatic outflow obstruction would carry exceptional risk; e.g. acute retention, urinary infection, and a raised blood urea would all double the operative mortality[6]. Today it is almost impossible to show that these hazards carry any significant extra risk[7], nevertheless it seems only prudent to avoid them if possible, and to offer operation before acute or chronic retention has supervened, and before the urine has become infected. There is a more practical reason to offer prostatectomy before the detrusor has failed, because the chronically distended detrusor will never function perfectly again[8].

Many attempts have been made to devise symptom scores, based on the patient's opinion of his own symptoms and how much 'bother' they give him[9,10] and these have been widely used in the evaluation of medical treatments for the prostate when the change in symptoms after the medication can be compared with those after the placebo. When these symptom scores are carefully tested against objective urodynamic evidence of obstruction they prove to be unreliable[11,12]. One symptom in particular, so long regarded as one of the classical features of 'prostatism', namely post micturition dribbling, is now realised to have nothing at all to do with prostatic obstruction[13].

For practical purposes the following is offered as a sensible policy for selection of cases for prostatectomy. In the early stages when the problem is that the patient complains of frequency, urgency, and the need to pass urine more than once or twice at night, an operation should be offered only when there is unequivocal urodynamic evidence of obstruction (see page 52). Even when there is obstruction, if the symptoms are mild, and there is no residual urine, the surgeon should continue to be cautious and consider postponing the decision for 6 to 12 months, waiting to see whether the symptoms improve and the outflow resistance lessens. It has been a constant finding in every study of a new treatment for the prostate that about one-third of men in this early category get better when given a placebo.

It is in this group of patients, especially the younger men with small glands, that one should consider using α-blockers. Not only may these give symptomatic relief, but a good response is a good sign that transurethral incision of the bladder neck will be successful.

The later features of significant residual urine, a hypertrophied and sacculated detrusor, diverticula or upper tract obstruction, all mean that the time for delay has passed. So too are any of the complications of residual urine such as infection or stone formation. When a patient develops acute retention after a crescendo of symptoms of outflow obstruction, this too should argue for operation.

There is one small group of patients who present with haematuria, and although the first priority is to rule out carcinoma of the kidney or bladder by the usual investigations, recurrent haematuria is very likely to take place and may give rise to painful clot retention if prostatectomy is witheld.

Clinical examination

Apart from evidence of chronic retention — the distended bladder, the wet trousers, and the smell of uraemia — early prostatic outflow obstruction gives no typical physical signs. Rectal examination cannot distinguish between urine in a bladder and a big benign prostate (Fig. 4.7).

(a)   (b)

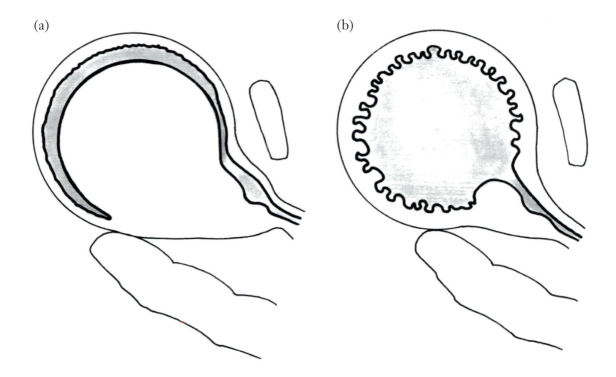

Figure 4.7
*Rectal examination cannot
distinguish (a) a big
benign gland from (b) a
thick walled bladder with
residual urine.*

Differential diagnosis

It is essential that the surgeon should take a careful history in the
traditional way, for no matter how careful a questionnaire may be,
and no matter how sophisticated the 'symptom score' that may be
calculated from it, certain important matters will not be brought to
light.

1. Anxiety

Anxiety is a common cause for frequency of micturition, which may
be very severe and exacerbated by urge incontinence. The tell-tale
features will only emerge in the course of taking a history, but
among them is the usual finding that the frequency occurs during
the daytime, and waxes and wanes according to the stresses of daily
life.

2. Depression

Many elderly men suffer from depression, and typically it wakes
them in the wee small hours when they get out of bed and empty the
bladder. Unable to get to sleep again, they may well have a cup of tea
or two, before trying to sleep, and before long they wake again to
empty the bladder.

3. Failure to concentrate the urine at night

Elderly people of both genders may secrete less pituitary antidiuretic hormone at night, while as they lie down, their vena cavae fail to contract and they continue to secrete the natriuretic hormone[14].

4. Bladder cancer

Not every patient with bladder cancer is aware of passing blood in the urine, and especially with carcinoma-in-situ the symptoms of frequency can exactly mimic those caused by early prostatic outflow obstruction.

Routine investigations

1. Uroflowmetry

This, the simplest and least invasive of all investigations will usually show a significantly impaired flow rate when there is outflow obstruction (Fig. 4.8). A very poor flow rate will be found whether the obstruction is from the prostate or a stricture and needs to be supplemented by other investigations.

Figure 4.8
Uroflowmetry.
(a) A normal flow rate.
(b) In prostatic obstruction.

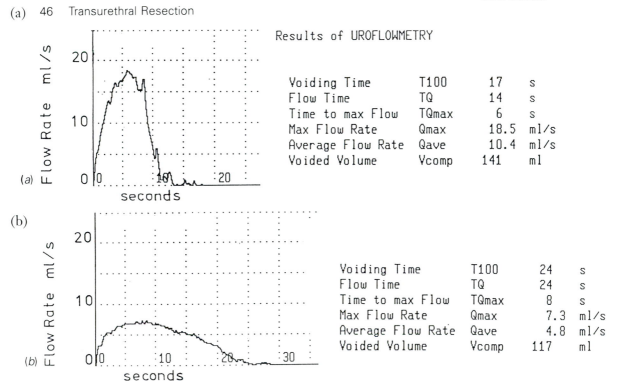

(a)   46   Transurethral Resection

Results of UROFLOWMETRY

Voiding Time	T100	17	s
Flow Time	TQ	14	s
Time to max Flow	TQmax	6	s
Max Flow Rate	Qmax	18.5	ml/s
Average Flow Rate	Qave	10.4	ml/s
Voided Volume	Vcomp	141	ml

(b)

Voiding Time	T100	24	s
Flow Time	TQ	24	s
Time to max Flow	TQmax	8	s
Max Flow Rate	Qmax	7.3	ml/s
Average Flow Rate	Qave	4.8	ml/s
Voided Volume	Vcomp	117	ml

Figure 4.9
Abdominal ultrasound showing trabeculated bladder with large middle lobe impression.

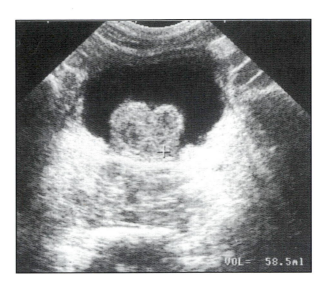

2. Ultrasound

Abdominal ultrasound scanning will detect enlargement of the prostate, trabeculation and sacculation of the detrusor, dilatation of one or both ureters, and can give a reasonably accurate measure of the volume of residual urine (Fig. 4.9). For practical purposes these two investigations are all that are needed, and they have supplanted the IVU except when there has been haematuria.

3. Urine cytology

Especially when there is a history of severe frequency, the urine should always be examined for malignant cells. Carcinoma-in-situ is a notorious mimic of prostatism.

4. Urine culture

The urine is always cultured so that appropriate antibiotic protection can be given to cover the operation.

5. Blood group

The haemoglobin and blood group are determined, and serum saved by the laboratory[15]. When preoperative investigations have discovered an unusually large prostate it may be wise to have two units of blood cross matched, depending on how quickly your laboratory can supply blood in an emergency.

6. Prostatic fibrinolysins

Abnormal fibrinolysins rarely occur from the presence of widespread metastases from cancer of the prostate: sometimes there is a warning in terms of spontaneous bruising or a history of unexpected bleeding. When in doubt the haematology laboratory should be asked to check for this and, if necessary, the operation is covered with a precautionary dose of cyclokapron.

Urodynamics

The only way to prove that there is outflow obstruction is by means of full urodynamic investigations. To get accurate and repeatable results the patient needs to have the pressure in the bladder recorded (Pves), for which a suprapubic line may be necessary: a rectal line records the intraabdominal pressure (Pabd), which is subtracted by a computer to give the pressure generated by the detrusor (Pdet). The bladder is filled and any uninhibited contractions of the detrusor are noted, which signify detrusor instability, and then the patient empties the bladder into a flow-meter, and the detrusor pressure is noted during the act of micturition[16] (Fig. 4.10).

Although for most practical purposes one can take it that any Pdet that is greater than 40 cm H_2O signifies obstruction, when a powerful detrusor has compensated for obstruction and gives a misleadingly high flow-rate, then one can have recourse to the useful nomogram of Abrams and Griffiths[17] which allows one to place the patient in one of three categories: obstructed, unobstructed or equivocal (Fig. 4.11).

Urodynamics of this quality are not available in every centre, and their interpretation requires skill and training, so that they should

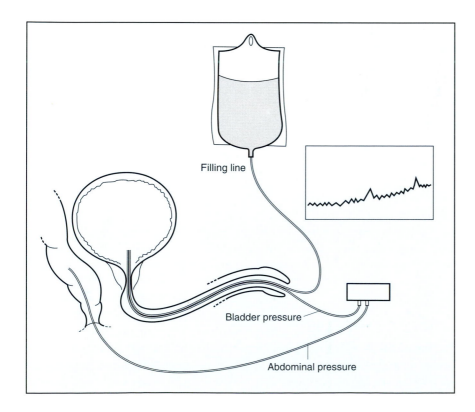

Figure 4.10
Set up required for urodynamic evaluation.

Filling line

Bladder pressure

Abdominal pressure

Figure 4.11
The Abrams-Griffiths nomogram.

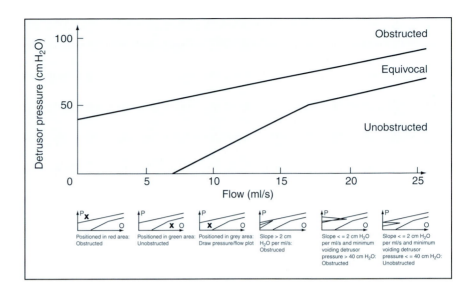

only be deployed when necessary. Their special value is in excluding men whose frequency is not due to obstruction, and in detecting those whose poor flow rate is not caused by obstruction, but by some weakness of the detrusor.

Shaving

There is no need to shave the skin before transurethral prostatectomy.

Anaesthesia

Many techniques of anaesthesia are suitable for transurethral surgery and a surgeon is wise to take more trouble over choosing an anaesthetic colleague than in telling him or her how to do their job. No particular technique is uniquely suited to endoscopic work. The requirements of the surgeon are that the patient should be still and free from pain. The field of operation should be uncongested, since venous engorgement increases the bleeding, so that CO_2 retention is to be avoided.

The patient must not grunt or cough, otherwise it is impossible to fill the bladder and keep a free flow of irrigating fluid, and without a free flow you cannot see what you are doing.

Excellent conditions are provided by inhalation anaesthesia with a mixture of nitrous oxide, oxygen and isoflurane, fluothane or ethrane. Deliberate hypotension is preferred by some surgeons but in our experience it is not the level of the blood pressure which is critical so much as the absence of congestion.

When the patient is particularly frail there are some advantages in spinal or epidural anaesthesia but for those with pulmonary insufficiency the anaesthetist can provide more oxygen with an inhalation technique. A caudal epidural in combination with general anaesthesia has much to commend it: the patient wakes without discomfort and there is none of the postoperative straining which sometimes causes reactionary haemorrhage.

Position on the table

Special tables adapted for endoscopic surgery have the advantage that they can be raised or lowered by the surgeon (Fig. 4.12). In many institutions, however, one must make do with the ordinary operating table, using appropriate supports for the legs. Many different types of support are available (Fig. 4.13), and the important thing is that the legs are kept in the correct position with the thighs making an angle of no more than 45° with the plane of the table (Fig. 4.14). To have the legs in this almost flat position puts less strain on the heart[18]. The so-called lithotomy position, as used in operations on the anus, produces an awkward angulation of the prostate as well as sometimes causing backache afterwards.

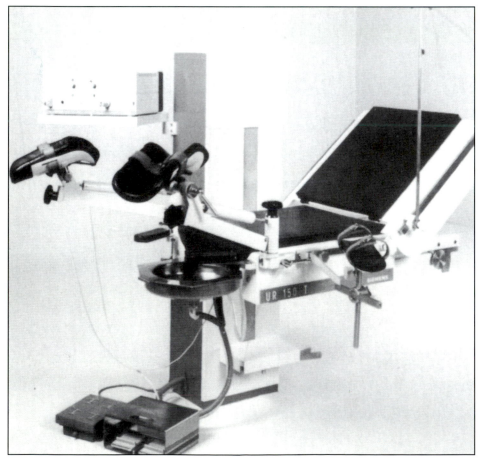

Figure 4.12
Siemens purpose-built operating table for transurethral surgery.

Figure 4.13
Adjustable Lloyd-Davies supports.

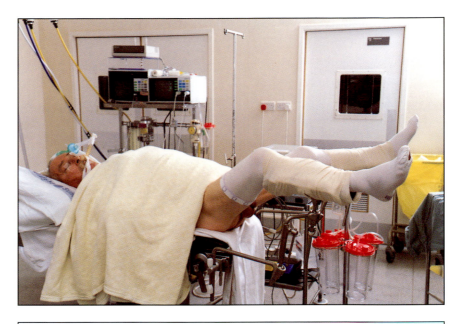

The wrong position for endoscopic surgery.

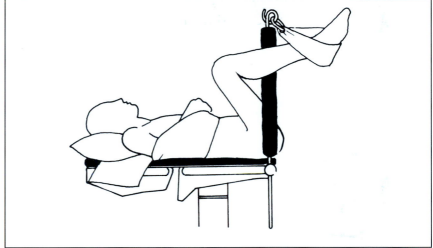

Figure 4.14
Mitchell slings, which allow the legs to be almost horizontal.

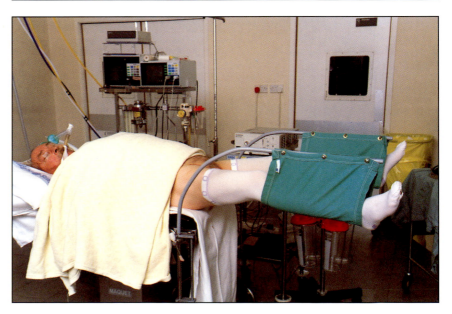

Diathermy pad

The earth pad is placed on the thigh, if necessary shaving a very hairy thigh. The appropriate safety devices should be checked to ensure that adequate contact has been made.

Skin cleansing

The skin of the genitalia and scrotum should be cleaned with a non-alcoholic antiseptic agent: iodine is avoided in view of the risk of causing a severe allergic reaction on the skin of the scrotum. The cleansing solution is applied with swabs held in forceps in the usual way. It is necessary to retract the prepuce and clean behind it.

Drapes

The legs are enclosed in roomy leggings or special disposable TUR drapes which are provided with a finger-cot to allow rectal examination during the procedure (Fig. 4.15). From now on the only surgically 'dirty' item in the procedure is the eyepiece of the telescope which makes contact with the surgeon's eyebrow or spectacles. This is a good reason for regarding the eyepiece or the TV camera as contaminated, placed on a towel reserved for it, and never handled by scrub nurse or surgeon.

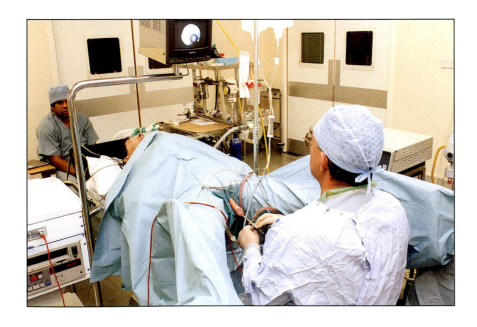

Figure 4.15
All-in-one drape for transurethral resection.

Preparation of the urethra

The urethra must be properly lubricated before introducing any instrument, and here the surgeon should borrow the usage of the engineer who always fills a cylinder with oil before inserting a piston into it. We use water-soluble gel containing dilute chlorhexidine: thereafter all the instruments are well 'buttered' with gel before being inserted. This is repeated whenever one feels the instrument dragging on the urethra.

Urethroscopy

After lubricating the urethra is it examined from end to end using the 0° telescope advanced under direct vision. This reveals a surprising number of soft annular strictures in the normal bulbar urethra. Once within the prostatic urethra care is taken to estimate the size of the gland and the distance from verumontanum to sphincter and to bladder neck. The sphincter is carefully identified.

Cystoscopy

The 0° telescope is now exchanged for a 70° telescope to examine the whole of the interior of the bladder. Special search is made for small tumours, especially those that may lie hidden behind the bump of the middle lobe, calculi that might need to be crushed and evacuated, and diverticula which must all be carefully examined to rule out stone or cancer.

Urethrotomy

Once the decision has been taken to go ahead with transurethral resection the 24Ch sheath is introduced. If the urethra is at all tight, an Otis or similar urethrotome is passed, and the urethra incised at 12 o'clock along its last 4 or 5 cm (Fig. 4.16). The urethrotome is passed with its blades closed, right into the bladder. Withdraw it past the external sphincter, open the blades to 30Ch in the mid-bulb, advance the knife and withdraw the instrument. If the urethra is examined after 6 weeks or so all that is left of the incision is a fine white line (Fig. 4.17).

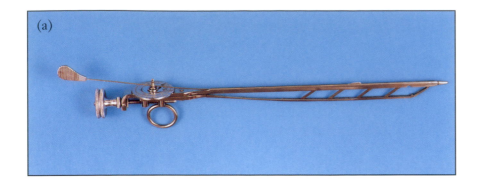

Figure 4.16
(a) Otis urethrotome.

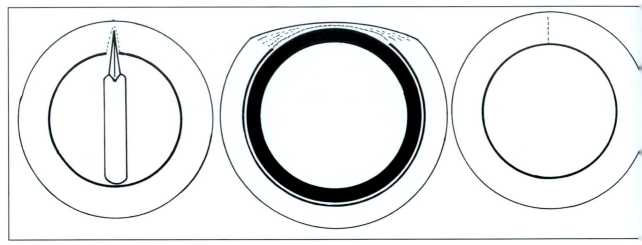

(b) *Clean incision of urethra.*   (c) *Large calibre sheath goes in easily.*   (d) *Heals without narrowing.*

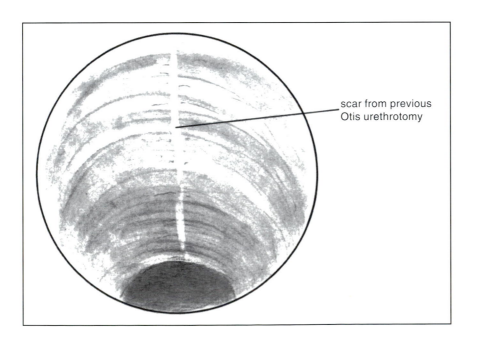

scar from previous
Otis urethrotomy

Figure 4.17
After a few weeks the site of urethrotomy is seen as a thin white scar, without any stricture.

The decision to perform an open enucleative prostatectomy

Today this is a rare operation in a urological centre, but when it is indicated there should be no hesitation in proceding to do it. The presence of multiple diverticula and large calculi is one good indication, for even if all the stones can be crushed, bits and pieces remain in the diverticula and can cause endless trouble afterwards.

Occasionally the patient suffers from some orthopaedic condition which makes it impossible for you to get your head between his legs, but the use of CCTV usually overcomes this difficulty.

What constitutes too large a gland is a matter of individual judgement. Incomplete removal of a little groove in the middle lobe is a waste of time, but occasionally an old man may able to pass water even when you have only been able to resect one lobe.

Occasionally, even though the prostate does not seem to be particularly big, the prostatic urethra is unusually stiff and rigid, and it is difficult to move the resectoscope or find one's landmarks. In these circumstances an open operation may be safer.

Severe bleeding from atheromatous arteries may be more safely and surely controlled by suture ligature at open operation, and an open operation may be more safe for the very large gland simply because haemostasis is so much more secure. Occasionally a patient will return with severe bleeding after previous transurethral surgery, and for these patients a retropubic prostatectomy may provide a more permanent cure.

In every case a number of factors have to be weighed by the surgeon; his or her experience with transurethral surgery, the need to avoid an abdominal incision and its attendant complications of pulmonary embolism and infection, and the difficulty of stopping bleeding when resecting a very large and vascular gland.

The big bloody gland of more than 100 g is, today, rather uncommon in the UK. It is easy to enucleate and haemostasis by suture ligature is exact and complete. With increasing use of preoperative ultrasound scanning, these very large glands can be detected ahead of time, and preparations made for an open operation in advance.

Whenever you have doubts, swallow your pride and perform an enucleative resection[19]. Never deceive the patient or yourself that you can always guarantee to do the prostate transurethrally. Make sure this is understood from the start. Let your fees be the same, and make sure that insurance companies understand that all methods of prostatectomy are equally deserving of reward.

One last factor deserves mention, for we surgeons are notoriously spendthrift of that irreplaceable commodity, our health. If you do much transurethral work, you will find yourself becoming far more tired than after an equivalent stint of open surgery. The intense concentration, the glare of the fibre-light, and the awkward way you have to bend your neck will make your eyesight suffer, and in time you may join the long list of urologists who suffer from cervical spondylosis[20]—a good reason for becoming adept with the use of the television monitor from an early age (see Chapter 3).

Informed consent

Certain things must be spelt out to the patient who is about to undergo a transurethral resection.

1. Sexual problems

Many of these elderly men are still sexually active, and it is necessary to discuss very carefully, and have written evidence of this, that there is a risk of retrograde ejaculation after operation, of the order of 50%, as well as a diminution in the sensation of orgasm, and a chance of erectile impotence which may be as high as 15%[21-23].

2. Incontinence

While the risk of incontinence is very low, slight stress incontinence is very common in the early weeks after transurethral resection, and it is wise to forewarn the patient about this. The risk of permanent incontinence is very low—perhaps about 1%, and opinions are divided as to whether there is any need to spell this out to a patient who may be anxious enough already[24].

3. Revision rate

The need to revise the TUR varies from one centre to another, but it is of the order of 15%, and this is something the patient needs to know about[24]. If explained in terms of the residual prostate continuing to grow, it is probably not far from the truth and easy for the patient to accept. But if it is not explained, and another operation becomes necessary in 5 or 10 years, the patient may be understandably aggrieved.

Antibiotics

There is no consensus as to the use of prophylactic antibiotics before transurethral resection except when there is clear evidence of urinary infection, or where there is a very high risk of urinary infection because the patient has been catheterised prior to operation. On the one hand, giving every patient antibiotics raises the chance of breeding multi-resistant organisms; on the other hand, positive blood cultures and the risk of septicaemia seem to be reduced by routine prophylaxis. The issues are debated by Hall *et al*[25].

Prophylaxis against pulmonary embolism

A careful audit of deaths occuring after transurethral resection revealed a surprisingly high incidence of pulmonary embolism, which might have been even higher had more post-mortem examinations been done[26]. As with prophylactic antibiotics there is no consensus among urologists. Subcutaneous heparin does not increase the risks of peroperative bleeding[27] and it has been shown that transurethral resection may safely be performed despite Warfarin treatment[28]. The subject is one that deserves far more research, and our practice is to use subcutaneous heparin in high risk patients.

References

1. McNeal JE. The prostate and prostatic urethra: a morphological synthesis. *J Urol* 1972; **107**: 1008.
2. Ahluwalia MS, Tandon HD. Nodular hyperplasia of the prostate in North India: an autopsy study. *J Urol* 1965; **93**: 94.
3. Green JSA, Bose P, Thomas DP *et al*. How complete is a transurethral resection of the prostate? *Br J Urol* 1996; **77**: 398.
4. McGuire EJ. The role of urodynamic investigation in assessment of benign prostatic hypertrophy. *J Urol* 1992; **148**: 1133.
5. Gosling JA, Dixon JS. Structure of trabeculated detrusor smooth muscle in cases of prostatic hypertrophy. *Urol Int* 1980; **35**: 351.
6. Blandy JP. Surgery of the benign prostate: the first Sir Peter Freyer memorial lecture. *J Irish Med Assoc* 1977; **70**: 517.
7. NHS Management Executive. *Prostatectomy for Benign Prostatic Hypertrophy.* Bristol: Health Care Evaluation Unit, 1992.
8. O'Reilly PH. The effect of prostatic obstruction on the upper urinary tract. In Fitzpatrick JM, Krane RJ (eds.) *The Prostate.* London: Churchill Livingstone, 1989; 111–18.
9. Riehmann M, Hansen BJ, Polishuk PV, Nordling J, Hald T. Symptom scores in benign prostatic hyperplasia. *Urology* 1997; **49**: 10.
10. Ko DSC, Fenster HN, Chambers K *et al*. The correlation of multichannel urodynamic pressure-flow studies and American Urological Association symptom index in the evaluation of benign prostatic hyperplasia. *J Urol* 1995; **154**: 396.
11. Hines JEW. Symptom indices in bladder outlet obstruction. *Br J Urol* 1996; **77**: 494.
12. Rollema H. Clinical significance of symptoms, signs, and urodynamic parameters in benign prostatic hypertrophy. In: Krane RJ, Siroky MB, Fitzpatrick JM (eds.) *Clinical Urology.* Philadelphia: Lippincott, 1994; 847–79.
13. Reynard JM, Lim C, Peters TJ, Abrams P. The significance of terminal dribbling in men with lower urinary tract symptoms. *Br J Urol* 1996; **78**: 696.
14. Nakamura S, Kobayashi Y, Tozuka K *et al*. Circadian changes in urine volume and frequency in elderly men. *J Urol* 1996; **156**: 1275.
15. Fraser I, Stott M, Campbell I *et al*. Routine cross matching is not necessary for a transurethral resection of the prostate. *Br J Urol* 1984; **56**: 198.
16. Hofner K, Jonas U. Urodynamics in benign prostatic hyperplasia. *Current Opinion Urol* 1996; **6**: 184.
17. Abrams PH, Griffiths DJ. The assessment of prostatic obstruction from urodynamic measurements and residual urine. *Br J Urol* 1979; **51**: 129.
18. Kedar S, Gaitini L, Vaida S *et al*. The influence of patient positioning on the hemodynamic changes in TURP patients with severe coronary disease. *Eur Urol* 1995; **27**: 23.
19. Blandy JP. *Operative Urology* 2nd edn. Oxford: Blackwell Science, 1986; 168–173.
20. Whitaker RH, Green NA, Notley RG. Is cervical spondylosis an occupational hazard for urologists? *Br J Urol* 1983; **55**: 585.

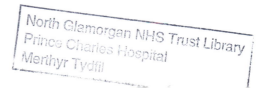

21. Dunsmuir VD, Emberton M. There is significant sexual dysfunction following TURP. Br J Urol 1996; **77**: 39.
22. Hanbury DC, Sethia KK. Erectile function following transurethral prostatectomy. *Br J Urol* 1995; **75**: 12.
23. Soderdahl DW, Knight RW, Hansberry KL. Erectile dysfunction following transurethral resection of the prostate. *J Urol* 1996; **156**: 1354.
24. Neal DE. Prostatectomy - an open or closed case. *Br J Urol* 1990; **66**: 449.
25. Hall JC, Christiansen KJ, England P *et al*. Antibiotic prophylaxis for patients undergoing transurethral resection of the prostate. *Urology* 1996; **47**: 852.
26. Lunn JN, Devlin HB, Hoile RW. *The Report of the National Confidential Enquiry into Perioperative Deaths 1993/1994*. London: NCEPOD, 1996; pp 181–2.
27. Wilson RG, Smith D, Paton G, Gollock JM, Bremner DN. Prophylactic subcutaneous heparin does not increase operative blood loss in transurethral resection of the prostate. *Br J Urol* 1988; **62**: 246.
28. Parr NJ, Lohn CS, Desmond AD. Transurethral resection of the prostate without withdrawal of Warfarin therapy. *Br J Urol* 1989; **64**: 632.

Chapter 5

The basic skills of transurethral resection

Just as in general surgery it is necessary to learn to make a clean incision with the knife, to tie a secure knot, to handle tissue with delicacy and to secure haemostasis with the minimum of trauma and tissue necrosis, so in transurethral surgery there are certain basic steps which the beginner has to master. Many of them can be learned on models and appreciated by watching a more experienced surgeon at work. Others can only be learned solo.

Cutting a chip

Cutting chips from prostate or bladder tumours can and must be practised before the beginner tries to resect in a live patient. Soap, or meat from the hospital kitchen, makes good tissue to learn on. The loop of the resectoscope cuts like a knife through butter without any effort: but it requires a little time to do its work. The cutting is carried out by a halo of sparks between the diathermy electrode and the tissues (see page 21). The cutting takes place without contact, but it takes a little time for the sparks to do their work. No force is ever required. The rate at which you work is limited by the rate of disruption of the tissues.

The shape of the chip is like a canoe (Fig. 5.1). It is as wide and deep as the loop, and its length is determined by the travel of the loop plus the extra length gained by moving the sheath in and out. There are two methods of cutting off the chip. The usual method is to sever the chip against the edge of the resectoscope sheath and for this reason many of the old masters such as Barnes insisted on a loop

Figure 5.1
The TUR chip is shaped like a canoe; it should be as deep and as broad as the loop, and as long as the travel of the loop in and out of the sheath plus the distance you move the sheath.

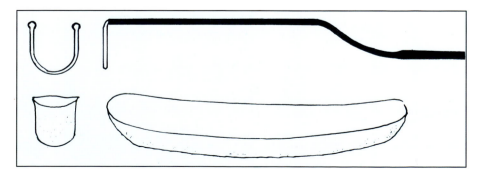

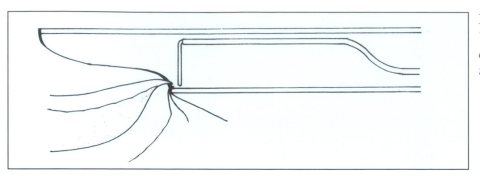

Figure 5.2
The usual method of cutting the chip off against the edge of the sheath.

which entered 1 or 2 mm inside the sheath[1] (Fig. 5.2). The second technique, advocated by Nesbit, was to bring the loop out completely before entering the sheath[2] (Fig. 5.3, 5.4).

If the loop goes too far inside the sheath sparks may damage the lens of the telescope and cause expensive damage, and for this reason some instrument makers design the loop so that it will not go inside the sheath. In practice, most urologists use the Barnes method, and will bend the loop: this is perfectly safe so long as there is still a gap between loop and lens (Fig. 5.5).

In time the edge of the sheath always gets more or less burnt away and when this is corrected by bending the loop the result can be disastrous (Fig. 5.6). The first rule, then, when starting to put the resectoscope together at the beginning of the operation, is to check the end of the sheath and the position of the loop. Send for an undamaged sheath even if this causes delay in the operation. A spare resectoscope sheath is a great deal cheaper than a new telescope.

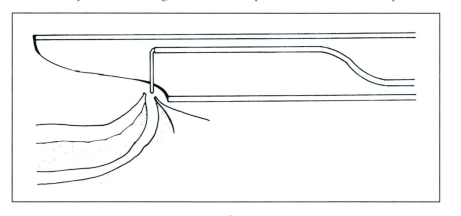

Figure 5.3
Cutting the chip off before the loop enters the sheath prevents any possible damage to the telescope.

Figure 5.4
Cutting a chip: (a) the loop is sunk into its full depth, (b) drawn towards you and (c) cut off before the loop enters the sheath.

(a)

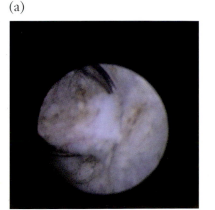

(b)

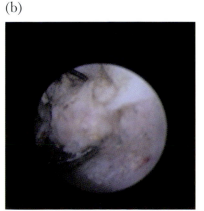

(c)

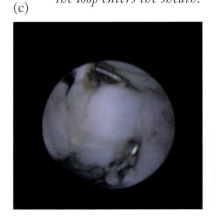

Figure 5.5
It is safe to bend the loop to allow it to enter the tip of the sheath so long as there is a gap between loop and telescope.

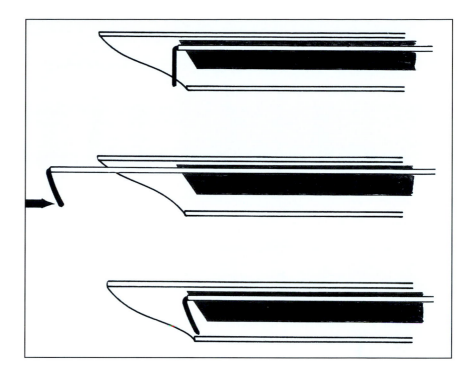

Figure 5.6
If the end of the sheath has been burnt away, and you continue to bend the loop, you risk damage to the telescope from the diathermy spark.

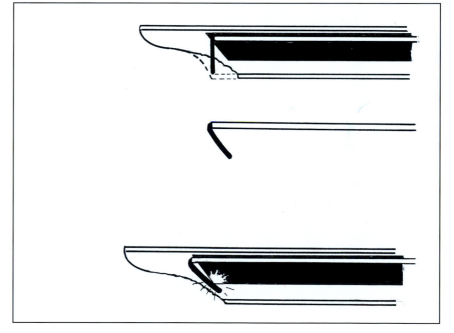

Rhythm

It is important to develop a smooth rhythm when performing transurethral surgery (Fig. 5.7). Begin by lifting up the handpiece to let the loop sink in as you start the stroke, and end by depressing it to lift out the loop. In a bladder tumour the action is similar although one must take care not to sink the loop too deeply into the wall of the bladder.

When resecting the bulk of the lateral lobes of the prostate, once the landmarks have been established, time is saved by making sure

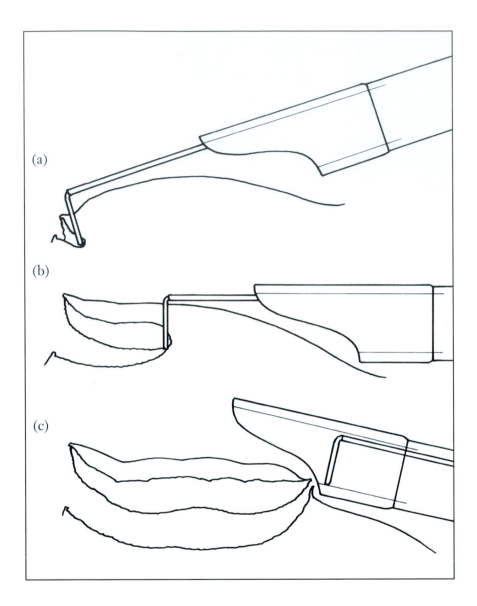

(a)

(b)

(c)

Figure 5.7
Cutting a chip: (a) lift the resectoscope to allow the loop to sink in, (b) keep it level as you cut the chip and (c) depress the sheath to cut off the chip.

that every stroke removes the maximum amount of tissue, i.e. the depth of the chip should be at least that of the loop and its length as long as that of the lateral lobe even if this means moving the sheath outwards, always making sure that you know the exact situation of the verumontanum.

If the electrode does not spark cleanly it will not cut, but will coagulate or char the tissue (Fig. 5.8). This is most likely to occur if you press the loop into the prostate instead of letting the sparks do the work. A crust of carbonized tissue may cover the loop. Clean it and start again.

If the loop does not cut at all, do not respond by asking for the current to be increased. Instead, carry out the following checks:
1. Make sure the loop is sitting firmly in its holder.
2. Check that the loop is not broken.
3. Check that the diathermy plate is securely attached to the thigh.

Figure 5.8
If the loop does not strike sparks it will cause deep local coagulation.

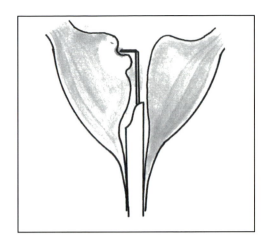

4. Check that the diathermy lead is attached to the machine.
5. Check the irrigating fluid: a common mistake is for the theatre team to hang a bag of saline instead of glycine.

If all these items have been checked and the loop still does not cut, you must change the diathermy machine. You cannot resect with a loop which merely chars: it drags in the tissues, makes it difficult to cut cleanly, and worse, risks producing a deep burn in the underlying tissues which may damage the sphincter (Fig. 5.9).

Figure 5.9
If the loop does not cut, check these causes of failure before asking for the current to be increased.

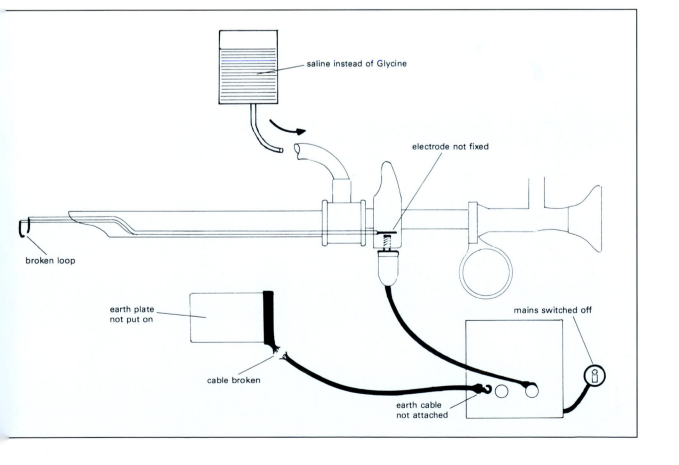

saline instead of Glycine

electrode not fixed

broken loop

earth plate not put on

cable broken

mains switched off

earth cable not attached

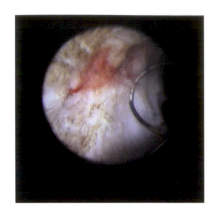
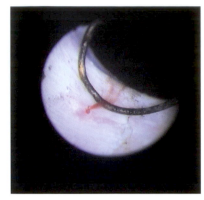
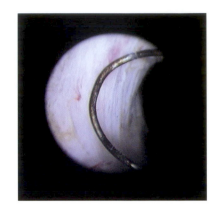

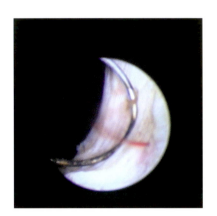
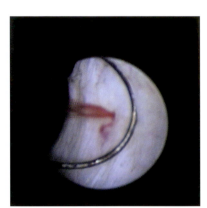

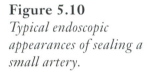

Figure 5.10
Typical endoscopic appearances of sealing a small artery.

Figure 5.11

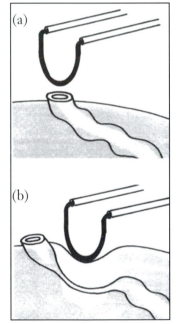

(a) A larger vessel may not be controlled by coagulating its mouth; the trick is (b) to squeeze the walls together by applying the loop just to one side to seal them with the coagulating current.

Haemostasis

Most of the light oozing which occurs during a resection comes from small veins which are cut as you resect the adenoma. This type of bleeding is minimized by using a continuous flow Iglesias irrigating system, but it should be stopped as you go along in order to keep a clear view. Any arterial bleeder should be controlled as soon as you see it by touching it with the loop and applying the coagulating current for a moment (Fig. 5.10). There is the typical noise of the coagulating circuit but there should be no charring or burning, only cessation of bleeding and a little whitening of the tissue.

When an artery is larger or thickened by atheroma it may be more difficult to close it off merely by touching its mouth. A useful trick is to compress the tissue to one side or other of the orifice of the artery (Fig. 5.11) so as to squeeze its walls together and allow the coagulating current to seal them.

Occasionally you will be misled by 'bounce' bleeding, when a fierce jet of blood rebounds off the opposite wall of the prostatic fossa: the appearance is easily recognized once it has been seen before (Fig. 5.12). The wily operator soon learns to turn his attention to the contralateral wall of the prostatic fossa to seek the true source of bleeding.

Figure 5.12
Bounce bleeding.

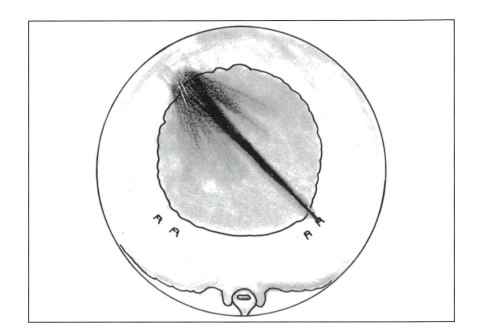

Figure 5.13
When an artery points straight at you all you can see is a red blur. The trick is to advance the sheath, tilt it to squeeze the vessel, and coagulate just upstream.

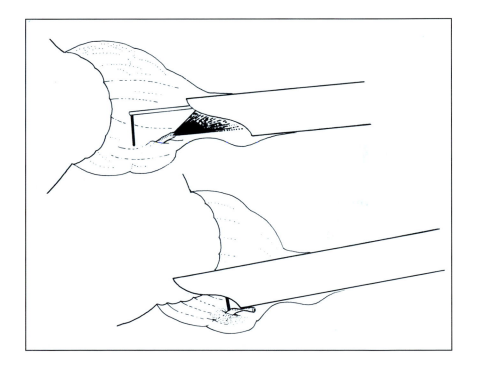

Another common source of confusion is the artery which is shooting out straight at the telescope. All you can see is a uniform red haze. The trick is to advance the resectoscope beyond the bleeder, angulate it to compress the vessel, and then slowly withdraw the sheath until the opening of the artery is betrayed by the emergence of a puff of blood (Fig. 5.13).

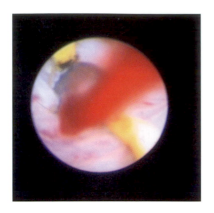

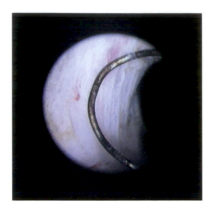

Figure 5.14 (left)
An artery bleeding straight at you. The roly-ball will coagulate it just upstream.

Figure 5.15 (right)
Coagulating with the roly-ball.

Coagulating just upstream of the artery will seal it off (Fig. 5.14). When you encounter large veins, multiple vessels set close together, or several atheromatous arteries which do not seal with the loop, change the loop for the roly-ball electrode (Fig. 5.15) and apply this sparingly to the source of the haemorrhage. Take care not to overdo the coagulation with the roly-ball: it produces heat at a depth which is proportional to the square of its diameter and invites late secondary haemorrhage.

Prophylactic coagulation

Sometimes it is obvious from the moment you pass the cystoscope that the resection is likely to be bloody. You can save yourself trouble by making a prophylactic attempt to control the main arteries before you start to resect. Using the roly-ball coagulate the prostate at 2, 5, 7 and 10 o'clock (Fig. 5.16) where the main arteries enter the gland. This simple measure minimizes subsequent bleeding, and may be repeated later on during the resection should bleeding recur.

Figure 5.16
Prophylactic coagulation of the main prostatic arteries at 2, 5, 7 and 10 o'clock.

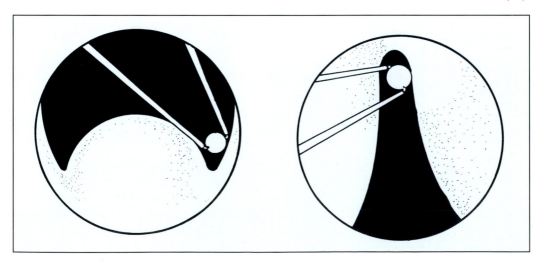

Veins

Veins are more difficult to detect than arteries, especially if the pressure of the irrigating fluid is equal to, or greater than, the pressure in the veins of the pelvis. For this reason you may see no venous bleeding at all during the resection, but as soon as the handpiece is removed there is a copious flow of blood.

Having sealed off all the arteries, the trick in finding the little veins is to slow down the inflow of irrigating fluid by adjusting the tap on the resectoscope until you can hardly see the tissue: little clouds of blood betray the position of the veins, which should be coagulated. It is worth taking time to go over the entire inner surface of the capsule at the end of the operation to seal them all. Time spent on this manoeuvre is time well spent.

Even so, there are some patients in whom, despite prolonged and patient haemostasis, there is still a copious ooze of venous blood. Here tamponade is effective. A catheter is passed on a curved introducer to make sure it does not catch under the bladder neck. Sterile water (40 ml) is injected into the balloon while it is well inside the bladder, and then the catheter is firmly drawn down so that the balloon compresses the neck of the bladder where most of the offending veins are situated (Fig. 5.17). Pull the catheter down, and maintain traction for 8–10 minutes, passing the time by

Figure 5.17
The Foley balloon is filled with 40 ml of sterile water (a) and pulled down to compress the veins at the bladder neck (b): traction is maintained by a gauze swab tied round the catheter and pulled back onto the glans penis.

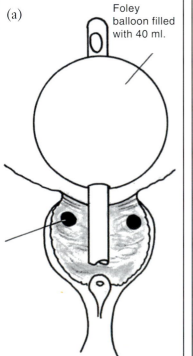

(a) Foley balloon filled with 40 ml.

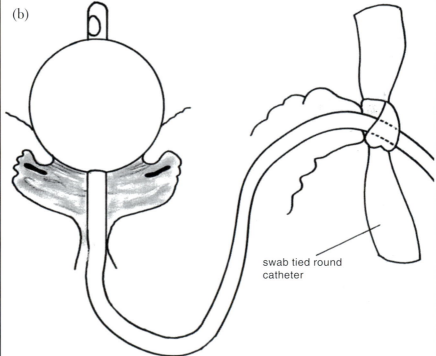

(b) swab tied round catheter

discussing politics or football with your anaesthetist. Often the bleeding will have been controlled. If not, keep it up by means of the Salvaris swab: two gauze swabs are tied moderately tightly around the catheter and pushed up against the glans penis. These swabs should be removed after 20–30 min lest a pressure sore be formed on the glans.

Never hesitate to reinsert the resectoscope if you have not properly controlled the bleeding, insist that the nurses do not clear away the trolley until you are satisfied that haemostasis is complete.

In the recovery room it is important that everyone is aware of the possibility of reactionary haemorrhage (see page 98). The hypotensive patient should be allowed to recover his blood pressure slowly and naturally. Aggressive restoration of the blood pressure in these old men with intravenous fluids or pressor agents may exacerbate bleeding and make things worse.

Evacuation of the chips

Every time you break the rhythm of resection to remove chips wastes time and one should keep the number of evacuations to the minimum, i.e. when the chips begin to fall back into the empty prostatic fossa and get in the way of the loop.

Of all instruments for removing clot and chips from the bladder the evacutor designed by Milo Ellik[3] is the most simple and effective (Fig. 5.18). Make sure that two of them are always filled and ready. Make sure also that you have mastered the knack of filling them and getting rid of all the air. The purpose of the bulb is to allow the irrigating fluid to go in and out of the bladder, to swirl it around and allow the chips and clot to float out of the bladder and fall down into the glass chamber. It must be used gently: if used roughly it is

Figure 5.18
Ellik's evacuator.

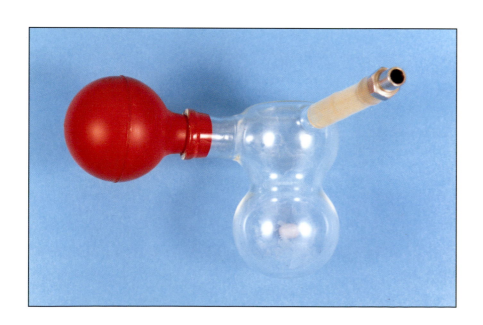

possible to rupture the bladder. Some surgeons prefer a wide nozzle hand syringe to the Ellik: readers should try for themselves. (Left-handed surgeons will find that instrument makers supply left-handed Ellik's.)

Keeping a clear view

Nothing is more important in resecting prostate or bladder tumour than being able to see what you are doing. There are many causes for a dim or obscured view, and some of them are worth mentioning for the beginner.

1. Bubbles on the lens may be caused by hydrolysis of the water by the electric sparks and cannot be avoided, but a more tiresome (and avoidable) source of bubbles can be traced to faulty connections of the tube and bag of irrigating fluid. The continuous flow resectoscopes minimize both types of bubble, but do not entirely avoid them (Fig. 5.19). When bubbles form, stop the flow of irrigant for a second and allow water to run out. If the bubbles persist, tap the telescope smartly in and out a few times.

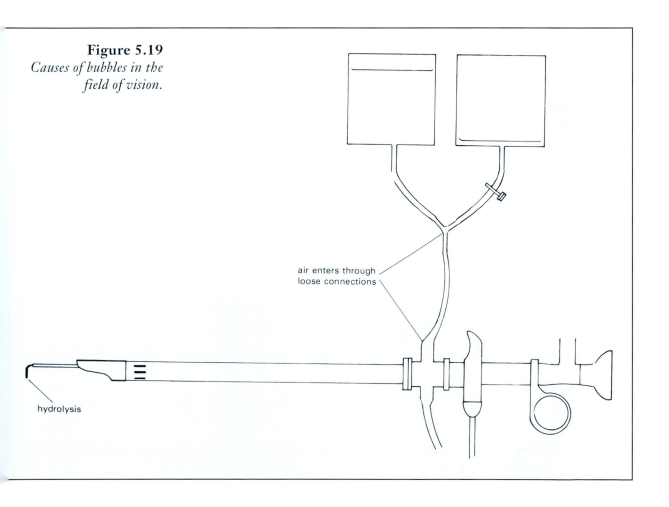

Figure 5.19
Causes of bubbles in the field of vision.

air enters through
loose connections

hydrolysis

2. A particularly irritating habit of the novice is to finger the eyepiece with a glove moistened with saline or lubricating gel. Others, given their first chance to look down the telescope huff and puff on the eyepiece. These lenses are made of soft optical glass and should only be cleaned with soft lint rather than cotton gauze which might scratch them. The best prevention is vigilance on the part of the surgeon and the application of the general rule that the eyepiece is regarded as surgically 'dirty'.

3. In conventional irrigating systems the most common cause for want of clear vision is obstruction of the water inflow (Fig. 5.19), usually because an inattentive nurse has let the bag run out. Sometimes the inflow becomes kinked or twisted. In continuous flow systems there may be imbalance between the negative pressure in the suction and the rate of inflow of the irrigating fluid. For this reason inflow and outflow taps must be under the control of the surgeon.

4. Whatever system of irrigation is used the inflow will stop when the bladder is so full that it can take no more. Since this means the pressure inside the bladder has risen, this is a state of affairs which should never be allowed to occur. This can occur with continuous irrigation, although it is much less likely to do so. If it does, the balance between inflow and outflow is wrong and must be adjusted. Most surgeons develop a sixth sense when the bladder is nearly full and when it is time to empty it out, and most resectoscopes begin to leak before this critical moment has been reached.

5. From time to time a chip of prostate or bladder tumour will be stuck to the lens or jammed between loop and sheath. In either case it is necessary to remove the handpiece. The lens should be cleaned using the jet of irrigating fluid or a piece of sterile lint. Blood that has been allowed to coagulate on the lens is a different matter. Use a broken wooden orange stick such as used for microbiological cultures: the wood does not scratch the optical glass.

6. If the telescope has gone misty, there is nothing you can do about it. Send for a spare and get on with the operation. The telescope will probably have to be returned to the manufacturer to get rid of water vapour.

References

1. Barnes RW. *Endoscopic Prostatic Surgery*. London: Kimpton, 1943.
2. Nesbit RM. *Transurethral Prostatectomy*. Springfield: Thomas, 1943.
3. Ellik M. A modification of the evacuator. *J Urol* 1937; **38**: 327.

Chapter 6
TUR technique for benign prostatic enlargement

Figure 6.1
The tissue removed during an enucleative open prostatectomy (a) is the same as that removed by TUR (b). In both, the inner zone adenoma is removed from the 'surgical capsule' of compressed outer zone.

Although several different techniques of transurethral resection have been described, their aim is essentially the same, to remove all the adenomatous tissue from the inner zone, leaving the compressed outer zone intact: the so-called 'surgical capsule'. The tissue which is removed during transurethral resection is therefore in theory identical with the tissue removed by an enucleative open operation[1,2] (Fig. 6.1). The various techniques of transurethral resection differ only in the order in which the bulk of tissue is removed. Two plans are described here: neither is in the least bit original and no particular preference is claimed for either. The important thing is that you should have a plan and stick to it, or else you will certainly get lost. Try each of these methods and choose the one which suits you best.

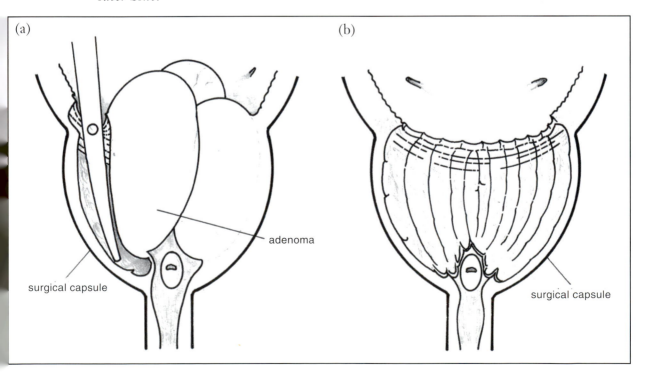

(a)   (b)

adenoma

surgical capsule

surgical capsule

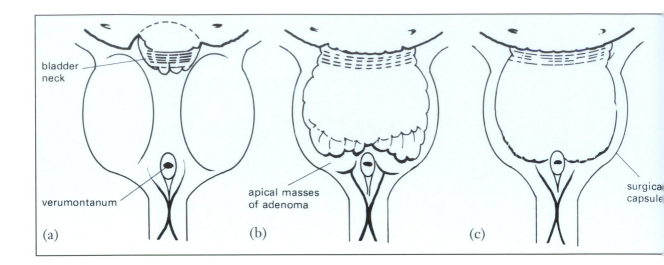

(a)   bladder neck   verumontanum

(b)   apical masses of adenoma

(c)   surgical capsule

In both methods there are three stages (Fig. 6.2):
1. Establishing the landmarks.
2. Removing the main bulk of tissue.
3. Tidying up.

In each method the resection begins with a preliminary urethroscopy and cystoscopy, careful lubrication of the urethra, and an internal urethrotomy if there is the slightest tightness of the resectoscope sheath (see page 57).

1. Establishing the landmarks

The landmarks in transurethral resection are the same whether you remove much tissue or only a little: the distal limit to the resection is the verumontanum, which stands like a lighthouse just proximal to that special region of the prostatic urethra which contains the supramembranous intrinsic component of the external sphincter (Fig. 6.3). This is a ring of elastic tissue, striated and unstriated muscle, quite distinct from and above the levator ani[3]. It is the essential part of the continence mechanism and must not be damaged.

Make sure you have seen the sphincter: bring the resectoscope out beyond it, cut off the water flow and see it contract like the anus in its characteristic way (Fig. 6.4). As you do this you will note an even more important feature: as the sheath of the resectoscope passes out beyond the sphincter it becomes instantly more loose. Recognizing this sensation is of great importance: it is as important as for the blind man to know what it feels like to step off the pavement onto the road. It is an instant warning that you are too far down the urethra for safety.

The proximal limit to the resection is the ring of muscle at the neck of the bladder. Having identified the verumontanum and the external sphincter, the next step is to find the ring of muscle at the bladder neck in the posterior middle line. The purpose of defining

Figure 6.2
The three stages of transurethral prostatectomy: (a) the landmarks are located, (b) most of the adenoma is removed, (c) the apical tissue is trimmed from either side of the verumontanum.

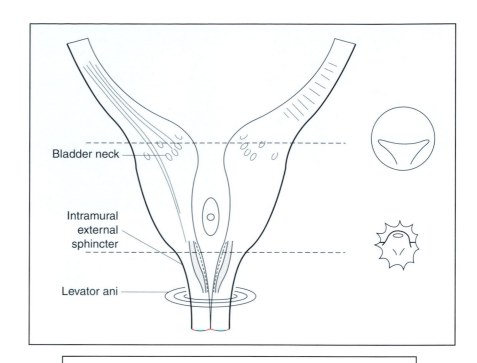

Figure 6.3
The three components of the sphincter mechanism of the bladder, bladder neck, intramural external sphincter (just distal to the verumontanum) and levator ani.

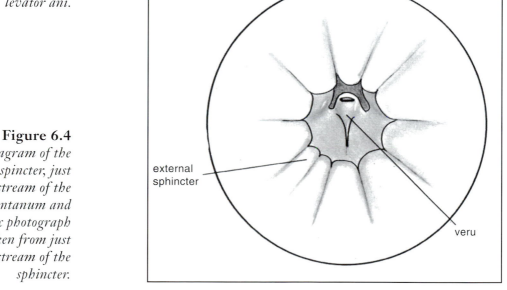

Figure 6.4
(a) Diagram of the external spincter, just downstream of the verumontanum and (b) endoscopic photograph taken from just downstream of the sphincter.

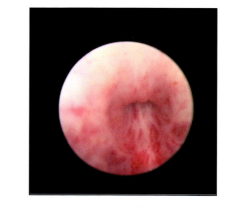

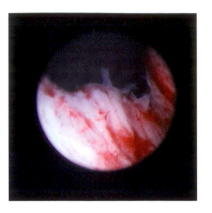

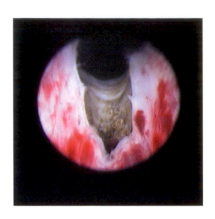

Figure 6.5
In a patient with a very small middle lobe the first cut reveals the transverse smooth muscle fibres of the bladder neck.

this proximal limit is to prevent you from inadvertently encroaching on the trigone and ureteric orifices. In some patients there is virtually no adenoma in the region of the middle lobe and the first loopful of tissue reveals muscle fibres immediately under the urothelium (Fig. 6.5). In others it is necessary to resect a considerable volume of adenoma before the bladder neck is exposed (Fig. 6.6). Once these fibres have been laid bare, they are left alone for the time being, even though it may be necessary to return to the bladder neck and trim more of it away at the end of the resection.

When the adenoma is very big the anatomy is distorted, and the lumps of adenoma in the apex of each lateral lobe extend well down below the verumontanum, distorting the supramembranous intrinsic component of the external sphincter (Fig. 6.7). When the time comes to resect this apical tissue great care is taken to lift it up with a finger in the rectum so that the loop does not cut the corner and injure the sphincter. It is equally important to refrain from coagulating in this region for fear of injuring the sphincter.

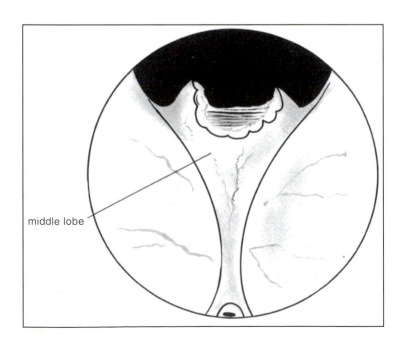

Figure 6.6
When there is a larger middle lobe more tissue must be removed before the bladder neck is exposed.

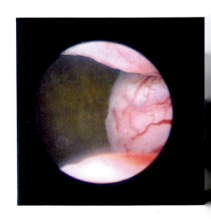

middle lobe

Figure 6.7
*In the small prostate:
(a) the verumontanum is
well upstream of the
sphincter, but in a big
bulky prostate
(b) the lateral lobe
adenomas bulge down past
the verumontanum and
distort the sphincter.*

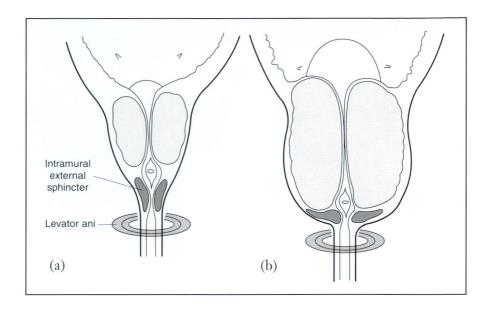

Having found the muscle fibres of the bladder neck, you now complete the removal of the middle lobe from the bladder neck down to just above the verumontanum (Fig. 6.8). You should now be able to see verumontanum and bladder neck in the same field of view and easily reorientate yourself if you get lost (Fig. 6.9).

The value of the verumontanum as a landmark is recognized by all experienced resectionists. In the old days of open prostatectomy it was not uncommon to see the verumontanum in the specimen, and the patients were not always incontinent because the intrinsic component of the external sphincter remained behind. But the verumontanum lies just upstream of the supramembranous sphincter and wantonly to remove it is not only to vandalize a useful landmark

Figure 6.8
*All the middle lobe tissue
should be removed from
the bladder neck down to
just upstream of the
verumontanum.*

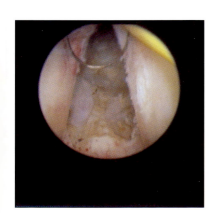

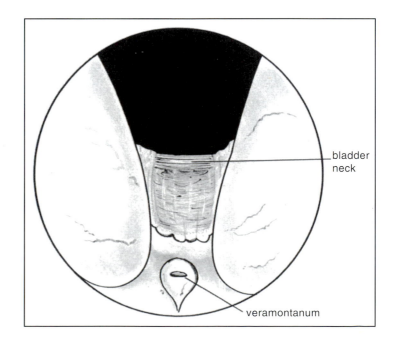

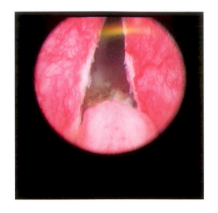

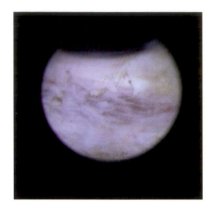

Figure 6.9 (left)
All the middle lobe is resected. You can see clearly from the middle lobe to the bladder neck.

Figure 6.10 (right)
Correctly resected middle lobe: there is a cobweb appearance under the bladder neck.

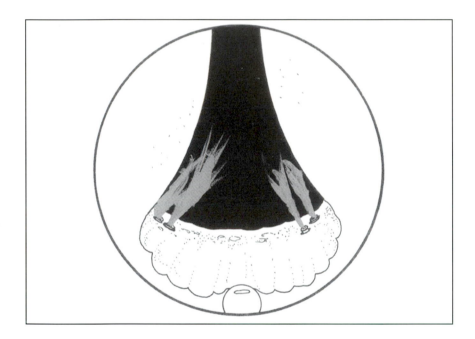

Figure 6.11
After resecting all the middle lobe, make sure Badenoch's arteries at 5 and 7 o'clock have been controlled.

which never causes obstruction to the flow of urine, but also to guarantee the end of any chance of ejaculation.

In the course of defining the bladder neck fibres it is not uncommon to create a small perforation under the edge of the trigone: there is a tell-tale appearance as if of a spider's web, and sometimes a distinct black hole in the connective tissue under the neck of the bladder (Fig. 6.10). By themselves these are not important, but they do mean you must take care not to pass the beak of the resectoscope under the trigone.

Once the middle lobe has been neatly cleaned out, take time to coagulate Badenoch's large arteries at 5 and 7 o'clock if these have not been completely controlled (Fig. 6.11).

2. Removing the main bulk of tissue

Keeping the landmarks in mind, the next stage of the operation is to remove the main bulk of adenoma.

1. First method

In the first method to be described, you rotate the resectoscope to bring the anterior commissure into view at 12 o'clock (Fig. 6.12). The object is now to liberate one of the lateral lobes from the capsule. Begin by taking one or two careful chips at 1 o'clock until the bladder neck fibres and the capsule is disclosed, remembering that the prostate is very thin anteriorly (Fig. 6.13). Continue to deepen the trench until the lateral lobe falls backwards into the defect left by removal of the middle lobe (Fig. 6.14). In doing this you may come across the little arteries of Flocks at 2 o'clock, which should be carefully coagulated[4] (Fig. 6.15).

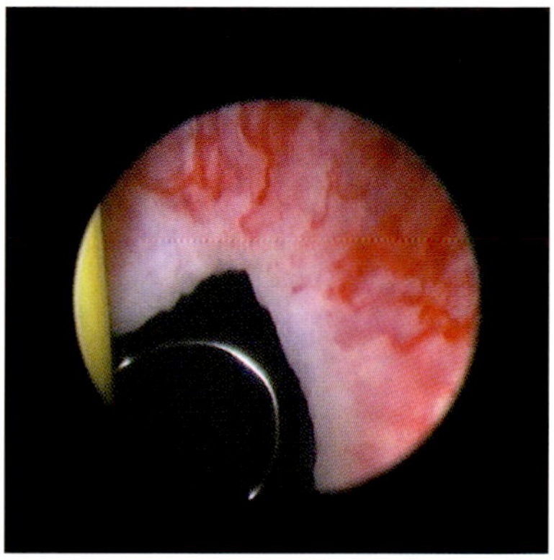

Figure 6.12 (left)
The anterior commissure.

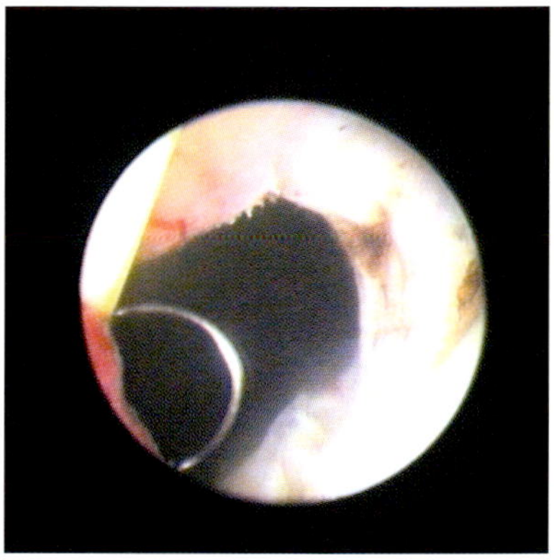

Figure 6.13 (right)
After the first one or two chips the capsule is exposed at 1 o'clock.

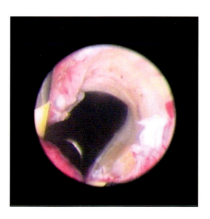

Figure 6.14
The trench is deepened and the left lateral lobe falls backwards.

Figure 6.15
The 2 o'clock arteries of Flocks need to be carefully controlled.

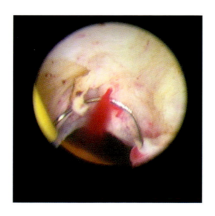
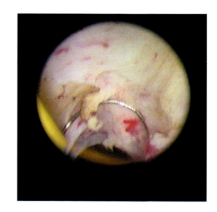

The next step is to remove the lump of lateral lobe which has fallen inwards and away from the capsule. Removing this part is usually relatively bloodless, because the main arteries have already been controlled at 2 and 5 o'clock. Trim the top of the lateral lobe away in a series of even cuts, keeping the surface flat (Fig. 6.16). Do not make the mistake of hollowing out the lateral lobe or you will find a thin shell of tissue will flop down and conceal the verumontanum (Figs. 6.17, 6.18).

Make sure that each stroke of the resectoscope loop cuts its chip off completely: do not make the mistake of leaving a chip attached at its distal end like a pine-cone (Fig. 6.19).

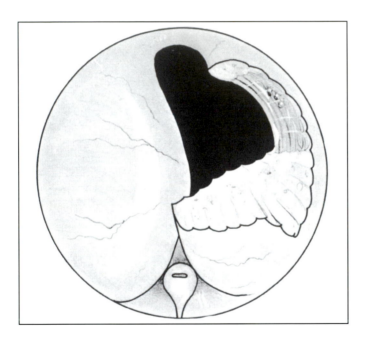

Figure 6.16
Trim the top of the lateral lobe evenly, keeping its surface flat.

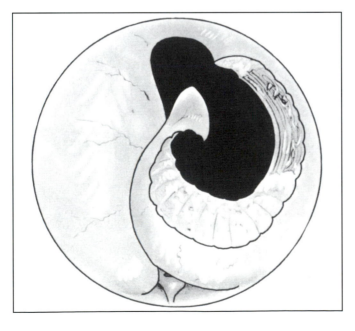

Figure 6.17
Avoid the mistake of hollowing out the lateral lobe and leaving a thin shell on the medial side.

Figure 6.18
Left lateral lobe hollowed out: the medial edge needs to be trimmed flat before it flops down and covers up the verumontanum.

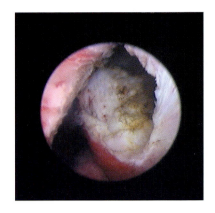

Figure 6.19
Make sure every chip is detached. Do not make a pine-cone of your resection.

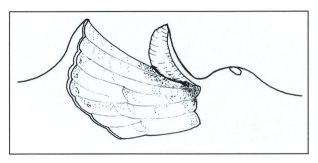

At this stage you can leave the most distal nubbin of apical tissue just near the verumontanum. Go over the whole of the inner surface of the prostatic 'capsule' from which you have removed the lateral lobe and make sure that all the bleeding has been stopped.

Check the position of the verumontanum and bladder neck, and then turn your attention to the other side. You will find that the anterior commissure seems to have moved and your original 2 o'clock trench seems now to be at 12 o'clock. Make a second trench (Fig. 6.20), detach the other lateral lobe, cut it away quickly and

Figure 6.20
Beginning the second lateral trench. Note that the anterior commissure seems to have moved over to the right.

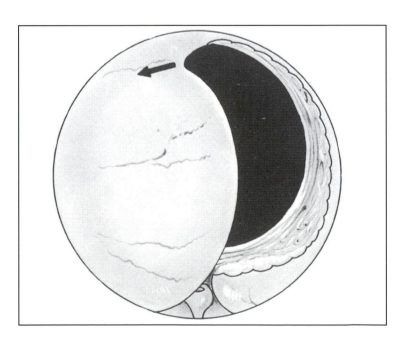

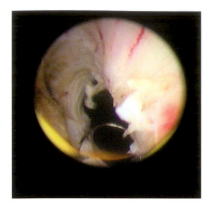 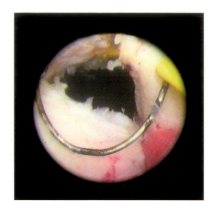

Figure 6.21
Beginning the resection of the right lateral lobe.

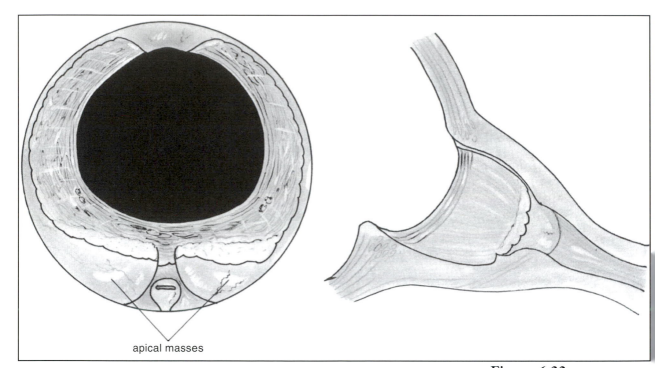

apical masses

Figure 6.22
Both lateral lobes are now removed, leaving only a little nubbin of apical tissue on either side of the verumontanum.

cleanly (Fig. 6.21), leaving only the nubbin of apical tissue adjacent to the verumontanum (Fig. 6.22). Go over the exposed 'capsule' and control the bleeding.

2. Second method

Many surgeons find it more comfortable to remove the bulk of the lateral lobes in one circular sequence (Fig. 6.23). After removing the middle lobe (as above) you start by taking one lateral lobe from the bottom upwards, across the commissure between the lateral lobes, and then down the other lateral lobe to the starting point. (Figs. 6.24, 6.25). It is important to start each chip at the level of the bladder neck and continue the cut down to the downstream limit of the adenoma, at the level of the verumontanum in order to maintain

Figure 6.23
RGN plan of resection: after removing the middle lobe, the operator starts at 7 o'clock and works all round the clock.

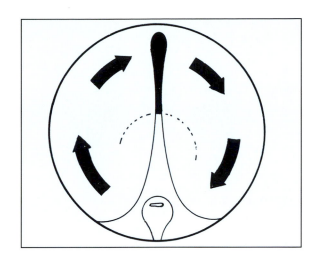

Figure 6.24
Beginning to resect the right lateral lobe, from 7 to 9 o'clock.

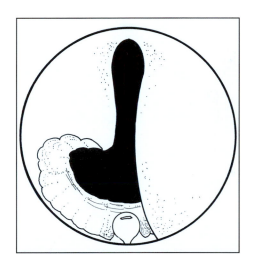

Figure 6.25
The right lobe is progressively resected from 7 to 9 o'clock.

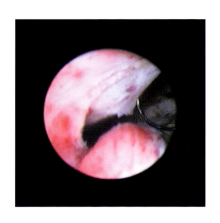
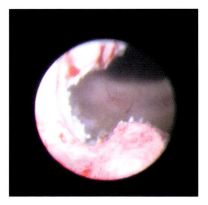
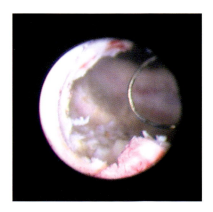

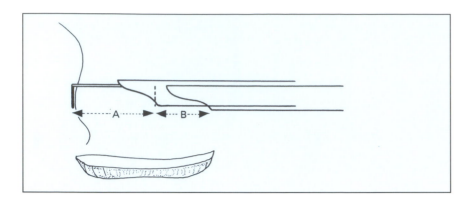

Figure 6.26
Long chips are made by adding movement of the sheath (b) to the movement of the loop (a).

Figure 6.27
Resecting the right lateral lobe.

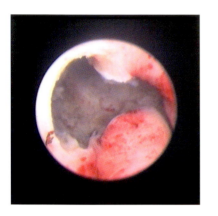
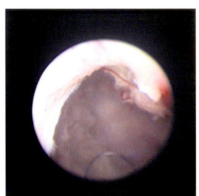
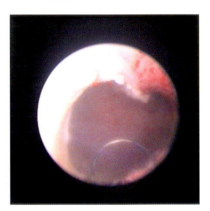

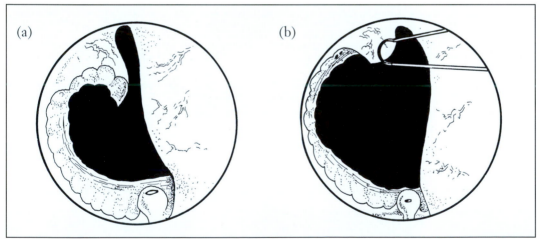

Figure 6.28
(a) Take care not to hollow out the lateral lobe.
(b) Near the commissure, where the adenoma is very thin, direct the loop laterally, not upwards.

a clear plan of progress. Long chips are achieved by moving the sheath in the urethra (Fig. 6.26). As you deepen the cut under the lateral lobe so the length of cut must be shortened to follow the barrel shape of the 'capsule'. (Fig. 6.27).

As your resection approaches the anterior commissure a mass of tissue will be seen hanging down. Remember again that the prostate is very thin here: do not hollow it out (Fig. 6.28) but trim it away with the loop pointing laterally rather than upwards. The 10 o'clock

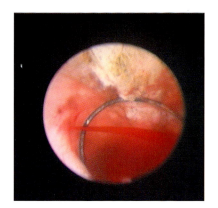

Figure 6.29
Flock's 10 o'clock artery will need to be coagulated.

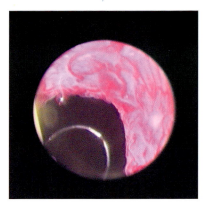

Figure 6.30
Continuing the resection across the anterior midline to the left.

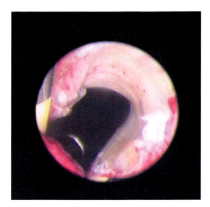

Figure 6.31
Continuing to resect the left lateral lobe, which has now fallen back.

arteries of Flocks will be found here and must be carefully coagulated. (Fig. 6.29).

The resection can then be carried across the midline at 12 o'clock bearing in mind that there is not much depth of adenoma in this part of the gland (Fig. 6.30). Continue the clockwise resection until the rest of the lateral lobe is removed (Fig. 6.31), sparing only the tissue adjacent to the verumontanum. .

3. Tidying up

In the third stage the apical tissue which has been left behind is removed very carefully. The danger here is that the sphincter may be damaged, and you do not start this part of the resection until you have completely controlled the bleeding and have a really clear view. Repeatedly check the position of the verumontanum and sphincter. Take only very short chips. It often helps to insert one finger in the rectum to lift up the verumontanum and offer the apical tissue to the loop rather than digging with the loop to scoop it out (Fig. 6.32). The finger in the rectum provides a very precise sensation of the amount of tissue remaining and of the nearness of the loop. Bleeding is seldom severe in the region of the apex and one should be very sparing in the use of the coagulating current.

After emptying the bladder, withdraw the sheath beyond the sphincter, and then gradually advance it: this will show where you have left adenoma behind. The usual places are just on either side of the verumontanum, and up at 2 and 10 o'clock. These are all carefully trimmed away (Fig 6.33). In removing the tissue adjacent to the verumontanum err on the side of caution. A gram or two of adenoma in this situation does not cause outflow obstruction, and a damaged sphincter can never be restored.

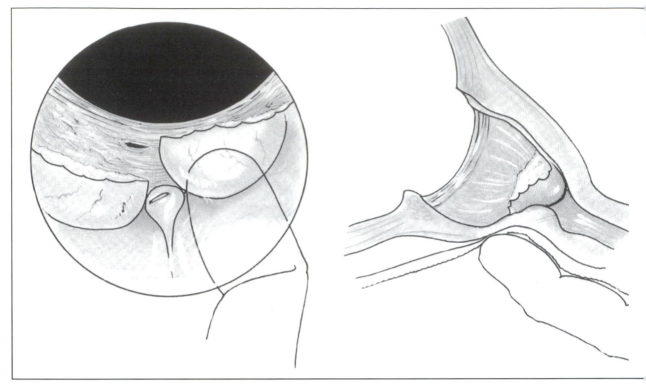

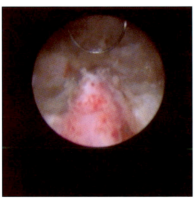

Figure 6.32
A finger in the rectum lifts the apical tissue up to the resectoscope loop.

Figure 6.33
Trim the apical tissue with great care to preserve the verumontanum.

Resection of the larger prostate > 50 g

Thanks to the instruments of today there is virtually no limit to the size of prostate that can be resected transurethrally so long as the surgeon can keep clearly orientated and maintain concentration and patience. It is unwise to attempt to resect a bulky gland when the resectoscope sheath does not slip easily over a huge mound of middle lobe, or when there is so much oedema and bleeding from the margin of the prostate that it is impossible to keep one's bearings. Such cases are uncommon, and it is interesting to see how seldom experienced resectionists need to perform an open prostatectomy. Be guided by your own common sense and judgement. Never be deceived by pride or by a sense of letting down your patient into embarking on a transurethral resection when you are not comfortable and confident: far better to do a clean, safe, open enucleative prostatectomy.

On the other hand, if you can see clearly enough to keep your bearings, it is hardly more difficult to remove 100 g than 40 g, since the steps of the operation are the same even though they take a little longer.

Stage 1

With a really bulky prostate there is much to be said for a preliminary coagulation of the main prostatic arteries at 10, 2, 5 and 7 o'clock using the roly-ball before taking out any tissue (Fig. 6.34).

In the first stage the middle lobe is often very bulky and bulges up and over the trigone (Fig. 6.35). It must be resected evenly along its top so that the mound is kept level and flat, otherwise it is easy to cleave it into two halves by a single deep channel in the middle

Figure 6.34
Prophylactic coagulation at 10, 2, 5 and 7 o'clock before starting to resect.

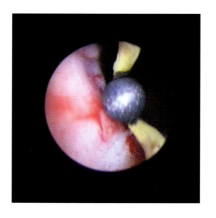

Figure 6.35
The middle lobe can be very large.

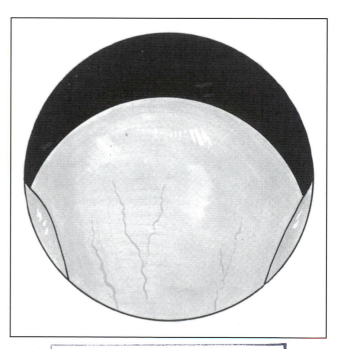

which leaves you bewildered and confused by what now seem to be two lateral lobes (Fig. 6.36). In removing the larger middle lobes the large 5 and 7 o'clock arteries will be exposed on either side and thoroughly coagulated (Fig. 6.37). It is wise to remove the whole of the middle lobe right down to within a few millimetres of the verumontanum. There is a tiresome tendency for a clot to sit just proximal to the verumontanum, making it difficult to see clearly. A finger in the rectum makes it easier to check on the position of the verumontanum and complete the resection of the middle lobe (Fig. 6.38).

As always, make sure of the haemostasis before going on to the next stage of the resection.

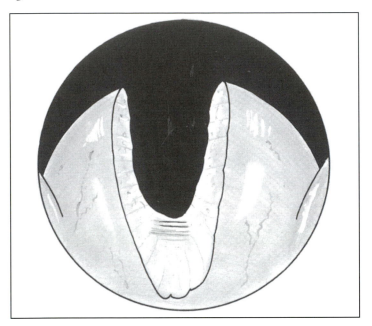

Figure 6.36
If you do not resect the middle lobe evenly you end up with a deep trench and 'two' middle lobes, which can be very confusing.

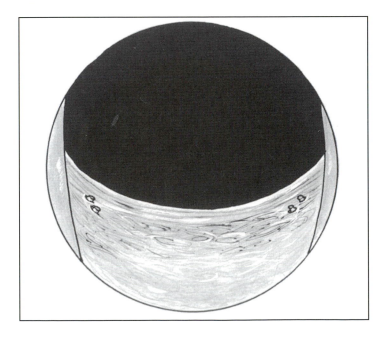

Figure 6.37
After resecting all the middle lobe, make sure the 5 and 7 o'clock arteries are completely controlled.

Figure 6.38
A finger in the rectum makes it easier to check on the position of the verumontanum.

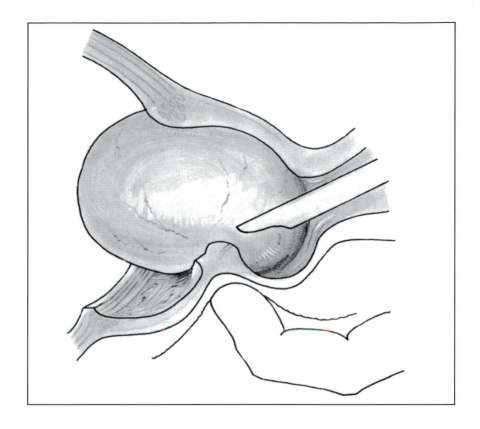

Stage 2

With large glands it is better to attempt to remove the whole of one lateral lobe than nibble away at both. If you prefer the first method, start the trench near the anterior commissure (Fig. 6.39), where the adenoma is always very thin, seal off Flocks' arteries, allow the

Figure 6.39
Start the trench near the anterior commissure.

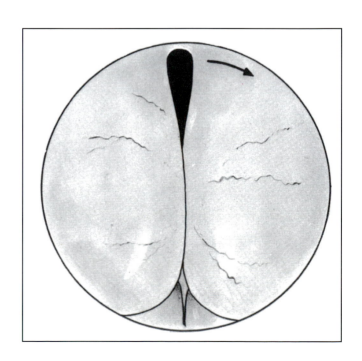

lateral lobe to fall down, and then cut it away with long even strokes, making sure you do not hollow it out (Fig. 6.40). A finger in the rectum will help to offer the adenoma to the loop rather than you having to dig into the barrel-shaped cavity of the capsule (Fig. 6.41).

If you take big long chips and move the sheath as well as the loop, you are less likely to create cliffs of unresected tissue half way down the prostatic urethra which may cause you to lose your bearings, but of course, you must not let the loop go past the verumontanum at this stage.

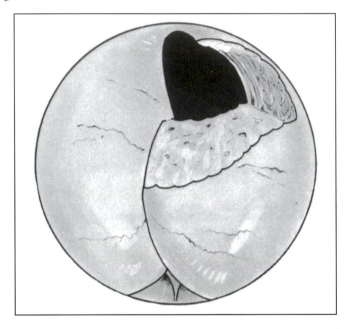

Figure 6.40
Trim the lateral lobe evenly and avoid hollowing it out.

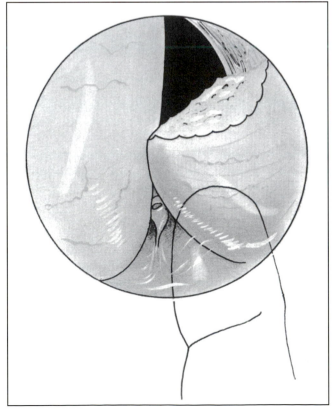

Figure 6.41
A finger in the rectum helps to push the adenome medially towards the loop.

Once the first lateral lobe has been removed, saving only the apical tissue (Fig. 6.42), go over the inside of the barrel carefully to stop all the bleeding; if necessary using the roly-ball. If you put off getting haemostasis at this stage you will find when you return that everything is confused by tenacious clot which conceals the origin of the bleeding. If there has been a considerable loss of blood, it is sensible to consider stopping the operation when one lateral lobe has been removed. The patient will often be able to pass urine perfectly well.

Figure 6.42
(a) Endoscopic and (b) lateral view after nearly all the left lateral lobe has been removed leaving only a small apical mass level with the verumontanum.

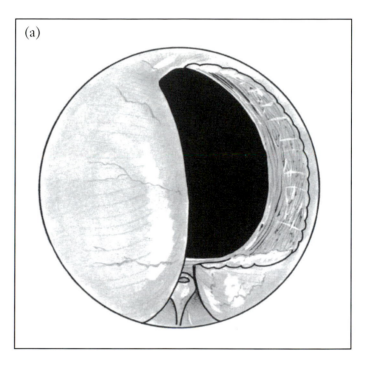

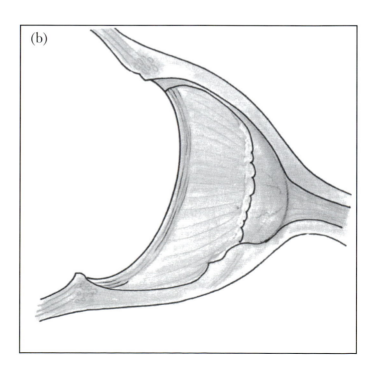

If all is well, go ahead and remove the other lateral lobe in the same way (Figs. 6.43, 6.44). It is of no importance which lobe you resect first but it is wise to get into the habit of doing things in the same order, a rule which is especially valuable when you are teaching others.

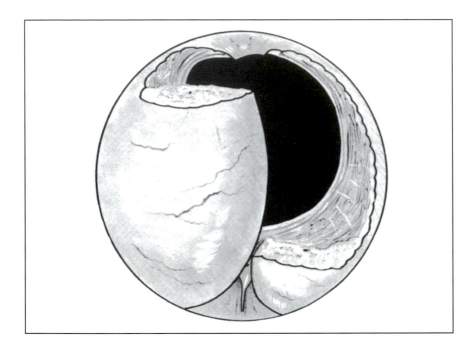

Figure 6.43
Removal of the right lateral lobe.

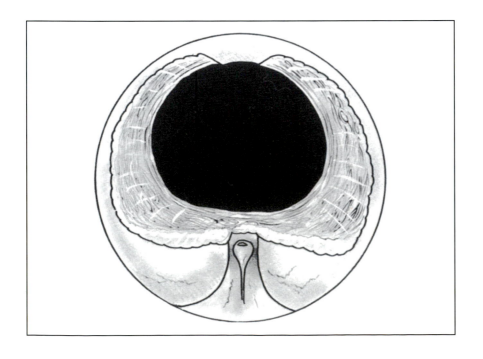

Figure 6.44
Both lateral lobes removed: apical tissue remains level with verumontanum.

The third stage in removal of a very large prostate is more difficult because the apical tissue often extends some way distal to the verumontanum (Fig. 6.45) where there is often a definite edge, 'Nesbit's white line' marking the distal limit of the adenoma[5]. The problem is to know how much of this has to be removed if all the obstruction is to be relieved, without risking damage to the sphincter.

Figure 6.45
(a) Endoscopic and (b) lateral view of a large prostate showing how the apices of the lateral lobe can extend downstream of the verumontanum.

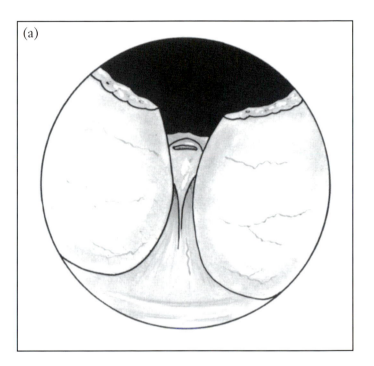

(a)

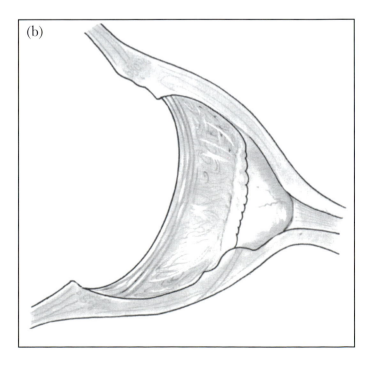

(b)

With a finger in the rectum to lift up the apical tissue, and taking very short bites with the loop, the bulk of the adenoma is trimmed away. A back-cut from just above Nesbit's white line helps to define the distal limit of resection. (Fig. 6.46).

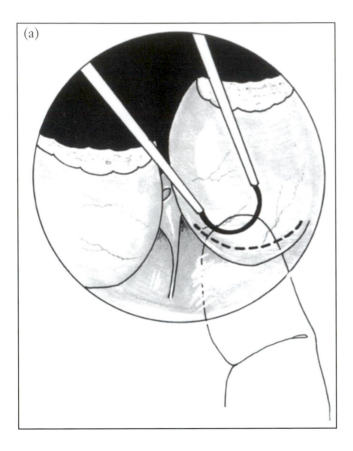

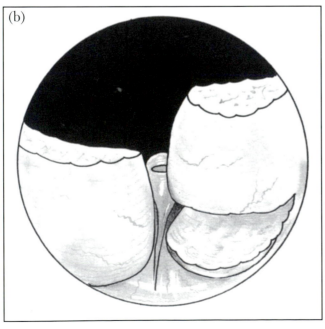

Figure 6.46
(a) A finger in the rectum lifts up the apex, well clear of the verumontanum.
(b) Short back-cuts with the loop define the lower edge of the apex.

Once the lateral lobes have been removed and the apices trimmed up, withdraw the resectoscope again distal to the sphincter and slowly advance it to identify any remaining tissue at 2 and 10 o'clock (Figs. 6.47, 6.48).

Figure 6.47
(a) First one and then (b) the other apices are cleared, leaving an intact verumontanum.

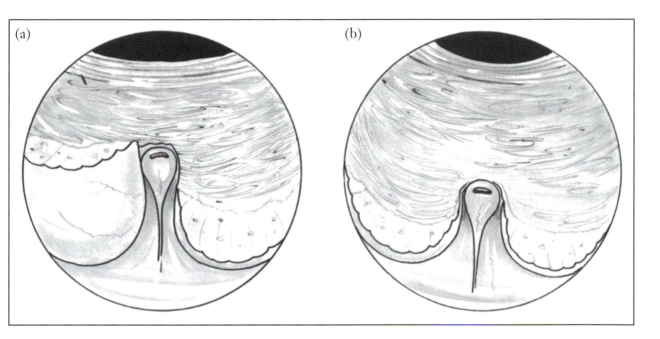

(a)

(b)

Figure 6.48
(a) The resection is complete: the verumontanum is intact, and (b) the cavity of the prostate has been clearly hollowed out.

(a)

(b)

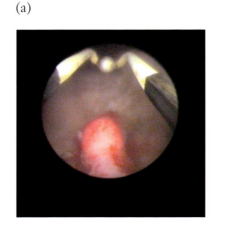 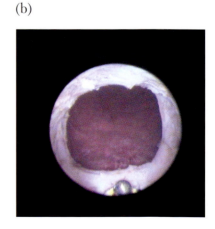

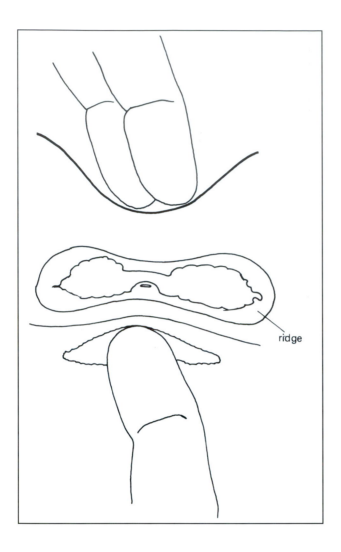

Figure 6.49
Bimanual palpation will reveal any lumps of prostate that have been left behind.

ridge

Finally, make a careful bimanual examination after emptying out the bladder. Usually all that is felt is a ridge of tissue on either side of the midline, exactly the same as after an enucleative prostatectomy (Fig. 6.49).

Perforations

Page[6] showed that the tissue remaining in the outer zone after removing the adenoma from the 'capsule' was composed of a compressed adenoma, which was in fact thinner than the loop of the resectoscope. There was no such thing as a true anatomical capsule, or at best only a paper-thin layer of connective tissue which was continuous with that which surrounded the vessels in the periprostatic fat. What we recognise as 'capsule' is in fact nearly a perforation. It is small wonder then that at the end of a resection it is usual to see little patches of fat (Fig. 6.50), and sometimes the dark

Figure 6.50
Capsule exposed, and a perforation showing fat globules.

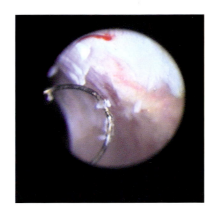 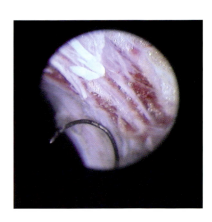

Figure 6.51
Deep perforation, probably the lumen of a vein.

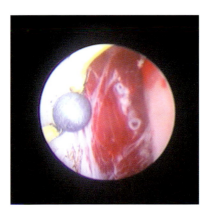

hole which is actually the lumen of a vein (Fig. 6.51). These little perforations are not dangerous and there is no need to drain the retropubic space even though there is always some extravasation of the irrigating fluid into it.

The same deep cut which has revealed fat may have damaged a large vein, which is not controlled by coagulation. In such an event the resection should be completed as quickly as possible and the bleeding controlled with tamponade (see page 71).

Perforations under the trigone

During the first stage of transurethral resection as the bladder neck is being exposed under the middle lobe it is very common to see small perforations which give the tell-tale appearance of a spider's web. By themselves these are not important, but there is a risk that the beak of the resectoscope may be driven inadvertently under the trigone, between the bladder muscle and the fascia of Denonvilliers.

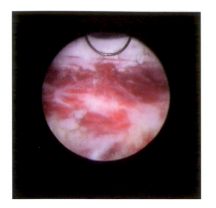 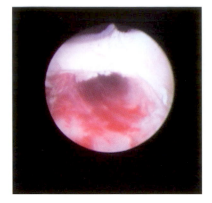 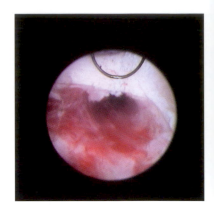

Figure 6.52
Perforation under the bladder neck.

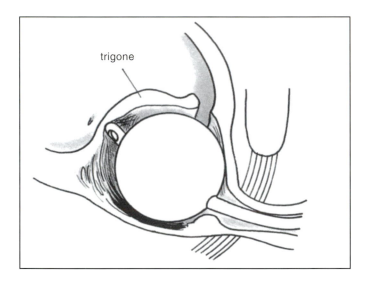

Figure 6.53
Inadvertent misplacement of the Foley catheter stripping up the trigone.

If this happens it produces a startling sight down the resectoscope (Fig. 6.52) but is not particularly dangerous: the danger is if the catheter is placed in this space and the balloon is inflated there (Fig. 6.53): hence the precaution of passing the catheter on an introducer.

Catheters and drainage

Whatever the size of the gland the operation is concluded by putting in a suitable catheter and arranging through and through irrigation (Fig. 6.54). It is not necessary to use a catheter larger than 22 Ch, but some surgeons prefer one made of PVC to latex. The irrigation is continued until the existing bag of glycine is finished, and then continued with saline. If the bleeding is more than a very faint pink the balloon should be filled with 40 ml and traction maintained (see page 71).

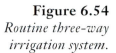

Figure 6.54
Routine three-way irrigation system.

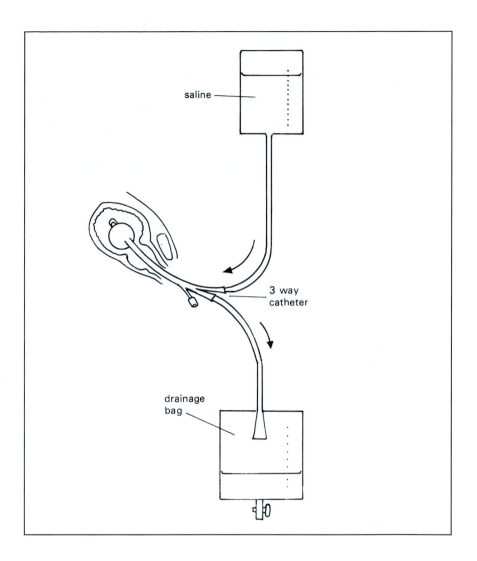

At this stage do not be in a hurry: have no hesitation in withdrawing the catheter and reinserting the resectoscope if haemostasis is not perfect. A few minutes of extra care at this stage may save hours of misery later on. If the patient has an endotracheal tube, wait for this to be removed, and for post operative coughing and straining to have stopped before allowing the patient to go to the recovery room.

In the recovery room the team should all know how important it is to keep the irrigation flowing and how necessary it is to summon the surgical team if the catheter is blocked. It is easy to irrigate or change the catheter in the recovery room, and when in doubt, the patient can be returned to the theatre for a second look.

The mildly hypotensive patient should be allowed to recover his normal blood pressure naturally, not by aggressive fluid replacement. Particular care must be taken with the bradycardiac hypotensive patient, a common enough situation after halothane anaesthesia. It may be better to correct the bradycardia with atropine rather than attempt to restore the blood pressure by fluids. A confused patient complaining of pain should be allowed to recover his senses, when rational discussion of the discomfort can often allay his unhappiness without the automatic recourse to morphine which may prolong the period of post operative recovery. The patient should only be allowed to return to the ward when the irrigation is running freely, is no darker than *vin rosé* and the patient is fully conscious.

Bladder neck dyssynergia

Younger patients may have outflow obstruction that seems to be caused by a failure of the α-adrenergic smooth muscle of the bladder neck to relax in synchrony with the contraction of the detrusor[7]. The predominant symptom is frequency, and urodynamics will show an abnormally high detrusor pressure and a poor flow-rate (see page 52). A therapeutic trial of α-blockers such as prazosin is given, and if the patient is relieved of symptoms, but dislikes the side effects of the drug, the option can be put to him of incision of the bladder neck. It is important that he fully understands the risk of retrograde ejaculation and the possibility of being rendered infertile.

After the usual urethroscopy and cystoscopy, an incision is made with a Collings' knife through the ring of bladder neck muscle. Classically the incisions were made at 5 and 7 o'clock but the proximity of the neurovascular bundles to the penis suggests that incisions at 2, 10 or 6 o'clock may be preferable[8] (Fig. 6.55).

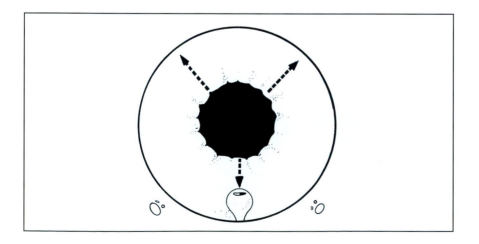

Figure 6.55
Bladder neck incisions which avoid the neurovascular bundles to the penis.

The small fibrous prostate

A different type of narrowing of the bladder neck is seen in patients with severe outflow obstruction but hardly any prostate to feel on rectal examination. They do not respond to α-blockers, and on resection the tissue is white and gristly and usually shows fibrous tissue on histological examination. Occasionally a more active granulation tissue is found in the specimen, in which case the patient should be carefully followed because recurrent stenosis of the bladder neck is then very likely. Mere incision does not result in an open bladder neck and it is better to perform a circumferential resection, leaving only a strip of mucosa in the region of the anterior commissure (Fig. 6.56).

Figure 6.56
Transurethral resection of a small fibrous prostate.

(a) First cuts.

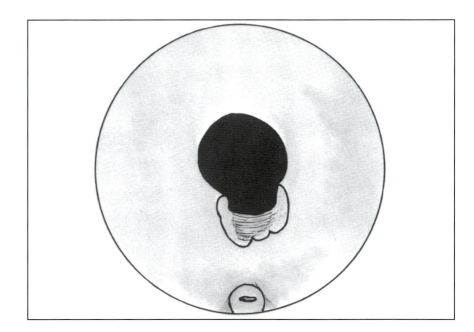

(b) Left half resected.

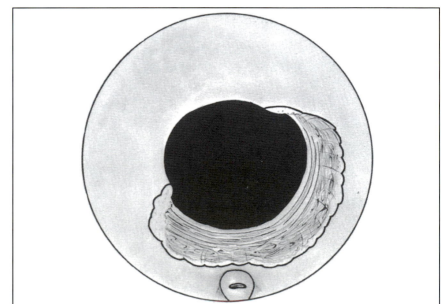

References

1. Green JSA, Bose P, Thomas DP *et al.* How complete is a transurethral resection of the prostate? *Br J Urol* 1996; **77**: 398.
2. Blandy JP, Fowler CG. Prostate: structure and function, in *Urology* 2nd Edn. Oxford: Blackwell Science, 1996; 363–74.
3. Gosling JA, Dixon JS, Humpherson RR. *Functional Anatomy of the Urinary Tract*. London: Gower, 1982.
4. Flocks RH. The arterial distribution within the prostate gland: its role in transurethral prostatic resection. *J Urol* 1937; **37**: 524.
5. Nesbit RM. *Transurethral Prostatectomy*. Springfield Illinois: Thomas, 1943.
6. Page BH. The pathological anatomy of digital enucleation for benign prostatic hyperplasia and its application to endoscopic resection. *Br J Urol* 1980; **52**: 111.
7. Caine M. Reflections on alpha blockade therapy for benign prostatic hyperplasia. *Br J Urol* 1995; **75**: 265.
8. Donker PJ, Droes JTPM, van Ulden BM. Anatomy of the musculature and innervation of the bladder and the urethra. In: Williams DI, Chisholm GD (eds.) *Scientific Foundations of Urology*. London: Heinemann, 1976; Vol. 2: 32.

Chapter 7

Transurethral resection of bladder tumours

Transurethral resection is the treatment of choice for all superficial bladder tumours that are not invading the detrusor muscle, or are not very anaplastic G3[1]. The resectoscope is used to take a biopsy and stage all tumours even where some adjuvant treatment is necessary[2].

Small tumours

When the tumour is very small it can be pinched off together with its base and a layer of bladder muscle with the sharp cup forceps. The base is then touched with the diathermy to stop any bleeding. An insulated biopsy forceps is available which can do both things without changing instruments (Fig. 7.1).

Figure 7.1
Insulated biopsy forceps.

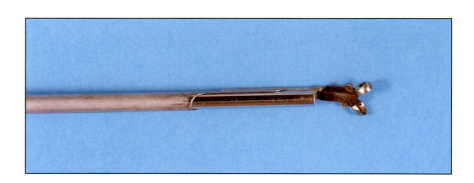

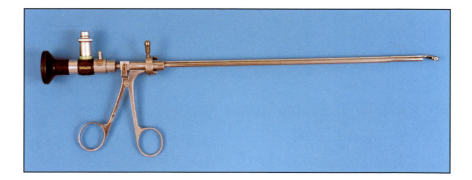

When there are multiple superficial tumours a few of them are removed in this way and the remainder coagulated with the roly-ball or Bugbee electrode (Fig. 7.2).

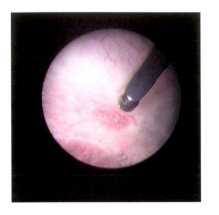 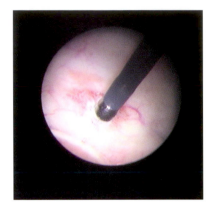

Figure 7.2
Very small tumours are easily coagulated with the Bugbee electrode.

Biopsy

After removing the obvious tumour, many surgeons routinely take small mucosal biopsies from apparently normal bladder (Fig. 7.3). The cup forceps are thrust at once into formalin to give histology free from the artefact caused by picking the biopsy off a gauze swab with a needle.

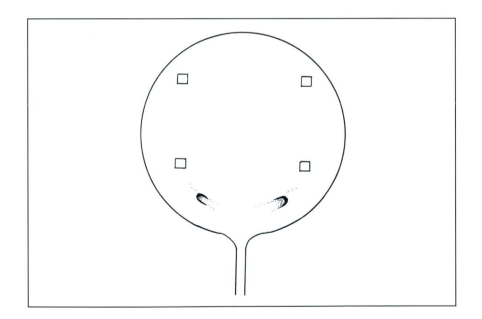

Figure 7.3
Random biopsies taken from the four quadrants of the bladder.

Mossy patches

Flat pink patches without obvious exfoliative tumour should be biopsied and then coagulated with the roly-ball electrode. When there is an extensive area of this superficial tumour the process can be speeded up by using the cutting current.

The average pedunculated tumour

The majority of superficial tumours are from 1 to 3 cm in diameter on a well-defined stalk. One or two large vessels can be seen entering the stalk from the adjacent mucosa. These tumours are too large to be removed with the cup biopsy forceps, but a single cut of the diathermy loop can often lift them off the bladder with a generous divot of muscle (Fig. 7.4), and the base is then thoroughly coagulated (Fig. 7.5).

Figure 7.4
Resection of a small papillary tumour, base and all.

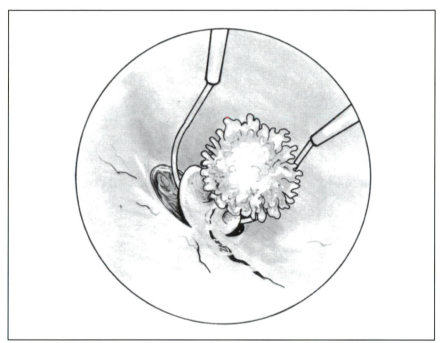

Figure 7.5
The roly-ball is used to coagulate the base.

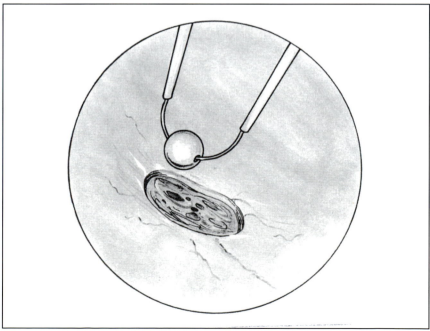

Larger papillary tumours 4–6 cm diameter

The first difficulty when resecting the larger papillary tumours with the conventional irrigating system is that the tumour seems to move away from the telescope as the bladder fills up, and you find yourself trying to hit a moving target. As soon as you start to resect the bleeding makes the vision even worse. This difficulty is very largely overcome by using the Iglesias type continuous flow resectoscope. If the inflow and outflow are correctly adjusted the tumour stays put and can be resected according to a methodical plan.

The second difficulty is that even though the stalk of the tumour may be quite narrow, the bush flops over and hides it, and until the big blood vessels in the stalk have been coagulated, resection of the bush is followed by more or less furious bleeding.

Do not attack the bush of the tumour as if you were trimming a hedge. Direct your attack at the stalk. It will probably be necessary to start by resecting the fronds of the bush which hide the stalk from you (Figs. 7.6, 7.7). As soon as you see the edge of the stalk, apply the roly-ball electrode to the stalk to coagulate it, and render the rest of the resection relatively bloodless (Fig. 7.8).

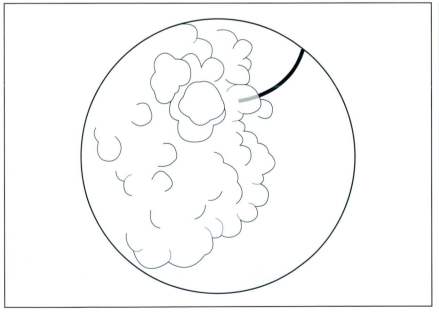

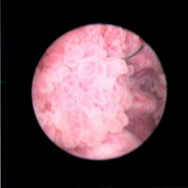

Figure 7.6
The first aim is to expose the stalk by resecting the overhanging bush.

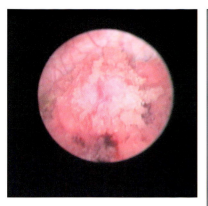

Figure 7.7
Overlying bush resected to reveal the stalk.

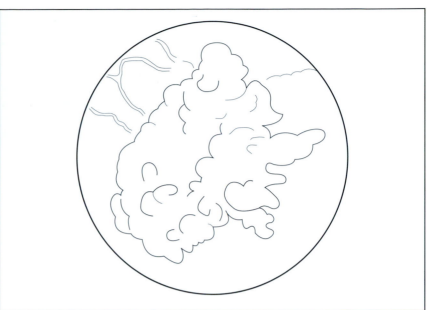

Figure 7.8
Once the stalk has been found, use the roly-ball to coagulate the main vessels.

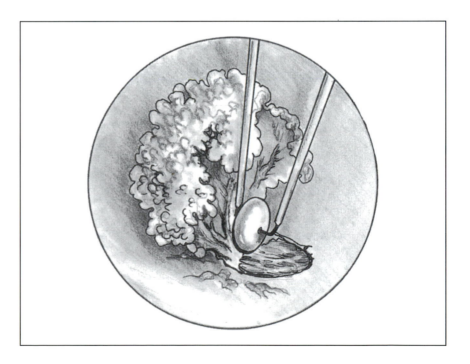

Then, having found the edge of the stalk, work round it, continuing to resect more and more of the overlying tumour until it has all been removed. Towards the end of the process you will find it easier to work from healthy bladder towards the stalk (Fig. 7.9). Finally, send pieces from the muscle in the base of the stalk for separate section to help the histopathologist establish how deeply it has invaded (Fig. 7.10). Make sure the tissue from the bush and the stalk are sent in separate specimen pots to the laboratory, labelled 'bush' and 'stalk' respectively. Finally, go over the base of the stalk thoroughly with the roly-ball electrode to effect haemostasis and

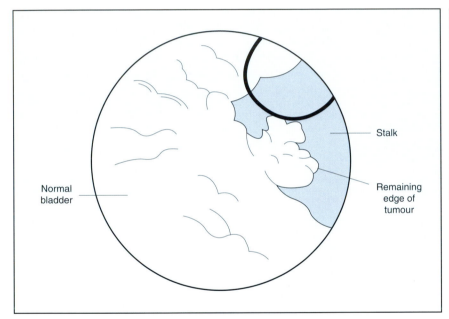

Normal bladder

Stalk

Remaining edge of tumour

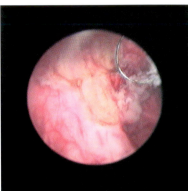

Figure 7.9
Trimming remaining tumour from the edge of the stalk.

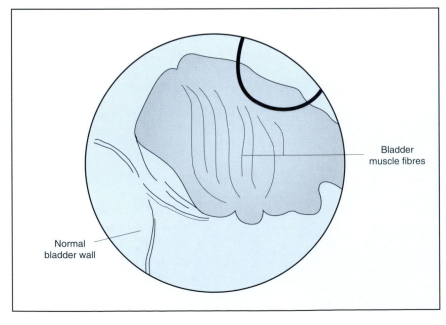

Bladder muscle fibres

Normal bladder wall

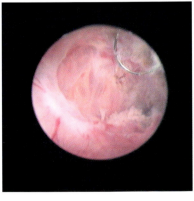

Figure 7.10
A separate biopsy, taken from the stalk, is sent to detect muscle invasion.

Figure 7.11
The base is coagulated with the roly-ball to achieve complete haemostasis.

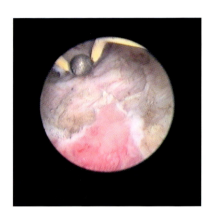

coagulate the layer of bladder muscle deep to your resection (Fig. 7.11). Haemostasis must be complete for unlike the prostate there is no way of effecting tamponade in the bladder.

After resection is complete, empty the bladder and perform a careful bimanual examination: induration in the wall of the bladder remaining after resection suggests invasion of muscle, and puts the tumour stage into T3.

Once haemostasis is complete, set up continuous irrigation as for a routine prostatectomy (see page 100).

Very large papillary tumours

Very rarely one encounters a group of giant papillomas that daunt even the most experienced resectionist. It is true that with the continuous irrigating cystoscope it is usually possible to resect them in the way described above, but occasionally the bleeding is so furious that it is impossible to see where to start. Here the Helmstein balloon can be useful, even though it is rarely needed[3,4]. The technique requires a very long period of continuous epidural anaesthesia because it relies on compression of the tumour by the balloon to produce ischaemic necrosis.

Under continuous epidural anaesthesia, which will produce a measure of hypotension, a large balloon is placed in the bladder tied to a catheter. Specially made and tested balloons are available for the purpose, but in the beginning Helmstein and others used ordinary toy balloons. The pressure inside the balloon is monitored continuously, as it is distended with glycine and the pressure is kept up for 6 hours (Fig. 7.12).

After the balloon is let down the ischaemic tissue of the tumour sloughs and an irrigating catheter may be necessary for the next few days until all the necrotic debris has come away. The bladder is re-examined after 3 weeks, by which time only the stumps of the previous tumours will be found. These are resected for staging in the usual way (Fig. 7.13).

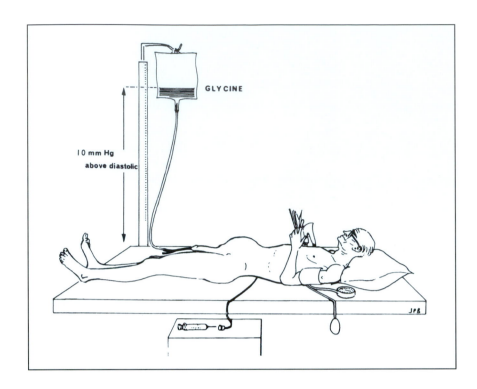

Figure 7.12
Helmstein's distension method.

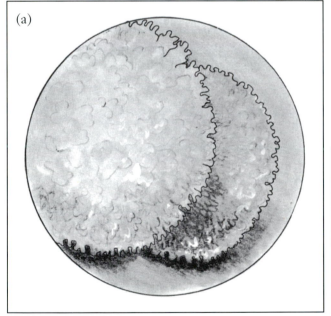

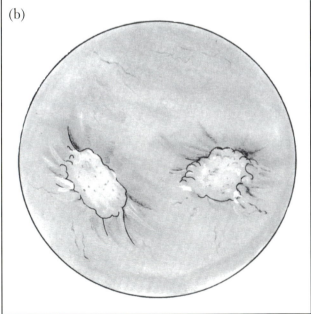

Figure 7.13
Three weeks after the Helmstein treatment, the bulky tumours (a) have sloughed away leaving only stumps (b) which are then resected.

Invasive solid tumours

When there is histological evidence of invasion of muscle the distinction between pT2 and pT3 is made according to the finding of induration on bimanual palpation after resection of the tumour is complete.

For those tumours which are obviously invading the bladder from the outset, it is not clear whether anything is gained by trying to resect all the exophytic tumour, although many surgeons feel that this controls bleeding and provides symptomatic relief from frequency and strangury, and many oncologists prefer that the bulk of the intravesical tumour should be removed, leaving less to be destroyed by irradiation. All agree that at the very least it is necessary to get evidence of tumour grade and stage, and this requires a good deep biopsy that reaches well into bladder muscle (Fig. 7.14).

Subsequent treatment of the G3 superficial tumours, and the muscle-invasive tumours of whatever grade, is a matter for controversy, the choice lying between total cystectomy, combination chemotherapy, radiation therapy, or some combination of all three: the matter is extensively debated elsewhere[5-7].

Figure 7.14
Large solid tumour: a deep biopsy which must include muscle, is taken from its edge for staging purposes.

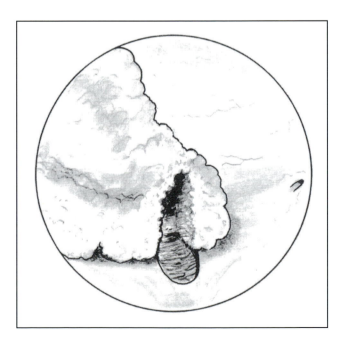

Adjuvant chemotherapy for superficial tumours

Every patient who has been treated for a bladder tumour will be carefully followed up by regular check cystoscopy, nowadays using the flexible cystoscope. There is considerable evidence that prophylactic adjuvant chemotherapy with Bacillus Calmette-Guérin, mitomycin, adriamycin and other agents will diminish the number of recurrences, and when multiple tumours are seen, or when they recur very frequently and in large numbers, these agents should be used[8–9].

Perforation

The bladder wall is often perforated during transurethral resection of a tumour and it is not uncommon to see the glistening globules of fat in the site of the stalk (Fig 7.15). As with the prostate, this is very seldom of any consequence so long as all the bleeding has been controlled. Extravasation of irrigating fluid is minimized by using a continuous irrigating resectoscope. The bladder should be drained.

The exception is when there is a tumour on the dome of the bladder and a deep resection of an invasive tumour has resulted in a perforation into the peritoneal cavity. This is very rare. It calls for laparotomy, not only to close the hole in the bladder and control bleeding, but also to make sure that any thermal injury to adjacent bowel is correctly oversewn or resected.

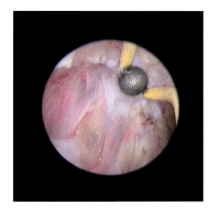

Figure 7.15
Perforation through the wall of the bladder into fat.

References

1. Jenkins BJ, Nauth-Misir RR, Martin JE *et al*. The fate of G3pT1 bladder cancer. *Br J Urol* 1989; **64**: 608.
2. Hermanek P, Sobin LH (eds.) *International Union Against Cancer. TNM Classification of Malignant Tumors* 2nd rev, 4th edn. Berlin: Springer, 1992.
3. Helmstein K. Treatment of bladder carcinoma by a hydrostatic pressure technique. *Br J Urol* 1972; **44**: 434.
4. England HR, Rigby C, Shepheard BGF, Tresidder GC, Blandy JP. Evaluation of Helmstein's distension method for carcinoma of the bladder. *Br J Urol* 1973; **45**: 593.
5. Gospodarowicz MK, Blandy JP. Radiation therapy for organ conservation for invasive bladder carcinoma. In: Vogelsang NJ, Scardino PT, Shipley WU, Coffey DS, Miles BJ (eds.) *Comprehensive Textbook of Genitourinary Oncology*. Baltimore: Williams & Wilkins, 1996: 513–22.
6. Lerner SP, Skinner DG. Radical cystectomy for bladder cancer. In: Vogelsang *et al*. (*ibid*): 1996: 442–63.
7. Splinter TAW, Scher HI. Adjuvant and neoadjuvant chemotherapy for invasive (T3-T4) bladder cancer. In: Vogelsang *et al*. (*ibid*) 1996: 464–71.
8. Morales A. Intravesical therapy of bladder cancer: an immunotherapy success story. *Jap J Urol* 1996; **87**: 93.
9. Witjes JA, Oosterhof GON, Debruyne FMJ. Management of superficial bladder cancer Ta/T1/TIS: intravesical chemotherapy. In: Vogelsang *et al*. (*ibid*) 1996: 416–27.

Chapter 8

Carcinoma and other disorders of the prostate and bladder

Carcinoma of the prostate

Since cancer usually arises in the peripheral zone of the prostate, when a small nodule is felt on rectal examination it is better to get tissue for histology by means of a transrectal biopsy, a procedure which today is most accurately performed under transrectal ultrasound control[1,2]. The later management of the small prostatic nodule is still a matter for debate which is beyond the scope of this monograph, and unfortunately is of little relevance to the large number of men who present at a stage when their cancer is not confined to the prostate, but is causing severe symptoms from outflow obstruction.

For these men transurethral resection of the prostate is but one incident in the management of their cancer, but at least to start with it is the one that is most necessary in order to relieve symptoms. The investigations and preparation are identical to those which apply to benign enlargement and the urethroscopy and cystoscopy are the same standard preliminary.

One difficulty is often encountered with prostatic cancer, where a carcinoma has made the entire prostate and prostatic urethra rigid, as if made of concrete, and it is difficult to pass the resectoscope. A helpful trick is to pass a filiform bougie, perhaps with a dog-leg bend at its tip (Fig. 8.1), to negotiate a tortuous pathway into the bladder. Once the filiform bougie is in place, an angled Timberlake obturator

Figure 8.1
A dog-leg bend on the end of a filiform bougie assists in getting it past a tortuous carcinoma of the prostate.

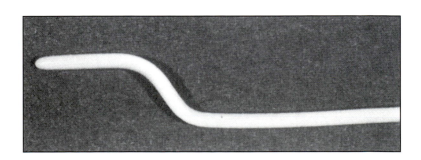

is fitted into the resectoscope sheath (Fig. 8.2), and the whole gently passed, following the filiform into the bladder. Once in the bladder, the tissue around the internal meatus is then resected, and at once the resectoscope sheath becomes mobile and the rest of the resection is straightforward.

If the angled Timberlake obturator is not available, the same procedure can be followed by passing the resectoscope sheath over a flexible Phillips follower which screws onto the filiform (Fig. 8.3).

In many cancers the landmarks may be difficult to find. Often the verumontanum is displaced or distorted by tumour, and sometimes the external sphincter is infiltrated by growth which makes it lumpy and rigid (Fig. 8.4). Since the cancer usually arises in the peripheral and caudal outer zone of the prostate and invades the capsule early on, you must not expect to find the usual difference in appearance between the 'bread' of the adenoma and the fibrous lacework of the

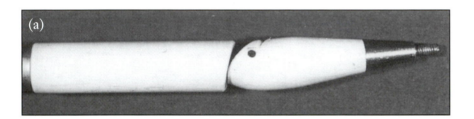

(a)

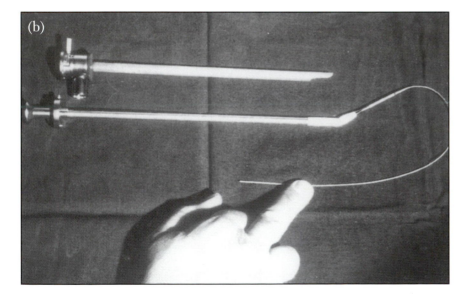

(b)

Figure 8.2
(a) An angled Timberlake obturator can be (b) screwed on to a filiform.

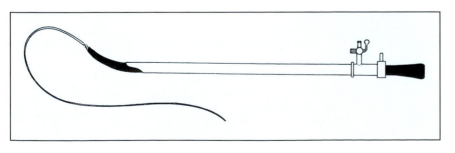

Figure 8.3
Alternative method of passing a resectoscope sheath through a hard, narrow prostate cancer using a flexible Phillips follower attached to the filiform.

Figure 8.4
The external sphincter and verumontanum are often distorted by carcinoma of the prostate.

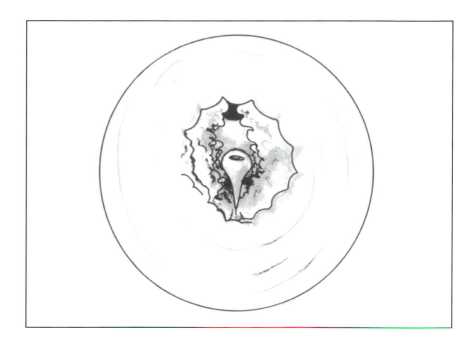

'capsule'. Instead the object of the operation is to carve an adequate funnel through the tumour from verumontanum to bladder neck (Fig. 8.5) through which the patient can pass urine. There is no point in attempting to do more. You should be extra careful when resecting in the region of the verumontanum and sphincter in the hope of preserving continence.

In resecting prostatic cancers it is particularly helpful to work with one finger in the rectum which will give a three-dimensional concept of the position of the resectoscope and the loop, even when the cancer has made the whole field stiff and unfamiliar.

Figure 8.5
In cancer the intention is only to carve a funnel-shaped cone from the bladder neck to the verumontanum.

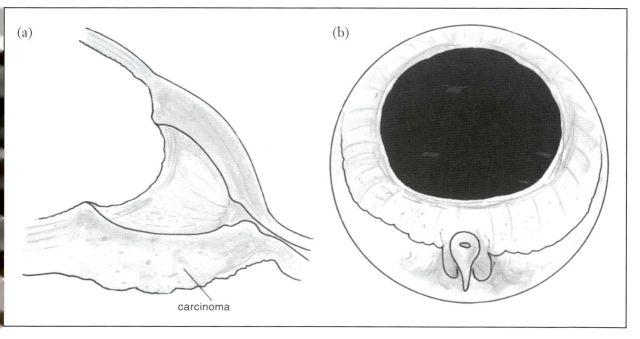

(a)

(b)

carcinoma

As a rule, bleeding is less profuse in cancer of the prostate, but one precaution should not be forgotten in men who present with widespread metastases, namely the possible presence of prostatic fibrinolysins which may prevent normal coagulation (see page 51). Be wary of this especially in the patient who gives a story of spontaneous bleeding and bruising.

It has been suggested on many occasions that transurethral resection might allow cancer cells to enter the circulation and so encourage dissemination of metastases. The evidence is disturbing, but inconclusive[3–4]. When the requirement is to confirm a diagnosis and establish the grade of the tumour, needle biopsies guided by transrectal ultrasound are more useful.

Calculi in the prostate

Small multiple calculi are so common as to be a normal component of the prostate[5] and they usually lie in the plane between inner and outer zones (Fig. 8.6), so that when they are reached in the course of transurethral resection of a benign gland it is a good indication that the 'capsule' has been reached and you have gone far enough. Sometimes the stones are so large that the loop of the resectoscope is broken when trying to dislodge them (Fig. 8.7)

Less common are the very large stones which protrude into the lumen of the prostatic urethra and sometimes extend up into the bladder. They are always half-covered by a layer of prostatic tissue (Fig. 8.8). This has to be resected before it is possible to push the stone up into the bladder, where it can be crushed and evacuated in the usual way[6].

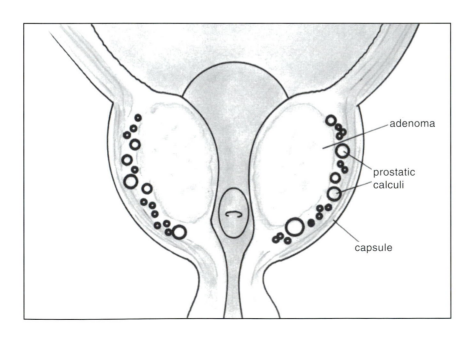

Figure 8.6
Small calculi are often found in the plane between the inner and outer zones of the prostate.

Figure 8.7
Larger calculi are revealed looking like eggs in a bird's nest, and may break the loop.

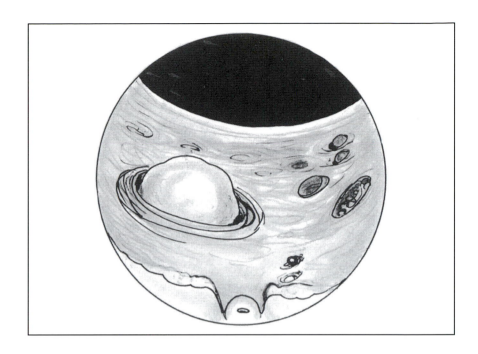

Figure 8.8
After uncapping the adenoma over a big prostatic stone it is pushed upwards into the bladder where it can be crushed and evacuated.

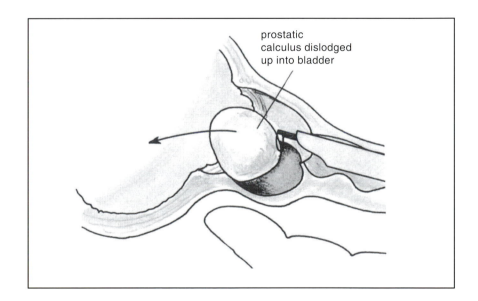

prostatic
calculus dislodged
up into bladder

Abscess of the prostate

Nowadays it is rare to see an abscess of the prostate, but it should always be suspected when a patient has fever, painful or difficult urination, and a very tender prostate on rectal examination[7]. Usually the prostate is more swollen on one side than the other. Sometimes the abscess bursts as soon as it is touched by the resectoscope; more often it is necessary to sink the loop of the resectoscope into the abscess, when pus pours out and the distended prostate collapses like a pricked balloon (Fig. 8.9).

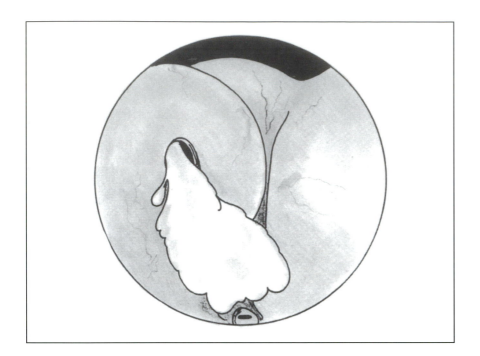

Figure 8.9
Opening an abscess of the prostate with the loop.

Chronic prostatitis

This is a diagnosis to be made with the utmost caution, and requires bacteriological confirmation by Stamey's method[8], and perhaps histological confirmation by biopsy under transrectal ultrasound control. Occasionally it is accompanied by outflow obstruction, which in these cases must be proven by urodynamic measurements (see page 52). Transurethral resection is likely to leave behind continuing infection in the residual outer zone tissue and relapse of symptoms is very likely to occur.

For the patient who complains of pain in the prostate and has no evidence of microbiological infection or the histological stigmata of inflammation, transurethral resection is contraindicated: it will almost certainly make the patient worse[9].

External sphincterotomy

In males with neuropathic lesions of the bladder an increase in the detrusor pressure may threaten the upper tracts; an incision of the bladder neck is often performed in the hope of allowing the bladder to empty at a lower pressure. In some cases however the external sphincter remains closed, and the dangerous increase in detrusor pressure persists. In such patients a deliberate incision of the external sphincter may be necessary so that the bladder will become incontinent, and the patient voids without any increase in pressure into a condom urinal.

The classical site for the incision into the external sphincter was at 5 or 7 o'clock, but to avoid injury to the neurovascular bundles of the penis the sphincterotomy incision should be made at 6 or 12 o'clock (Fig. 8.10).

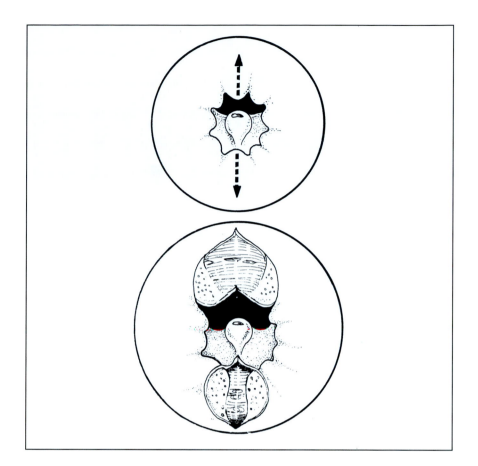

Figure 8.10
Sphincterotomy. Midline incisions avoid the neurovascular bundles to the penis.

Bladder calculi

Small stones are often found behind enlarged prostates. There are few calculi which cannot be crushed and evacuated. A number of instruments are now available for crushing bladder calculi including the optical lithotrite (Fig. 8.11), stone-crushing forceps (Fig. 8.12) and Mauermayer's stone punch (Fig. 8.13).

These optical instruments are ideal for small calculi, and allow the stone to be broken up under vision and evacuated with an Ellik evacuator (Fig. 8.14).

Figure 8.11
Storz optical lithotrite.

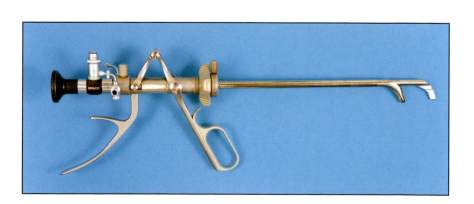

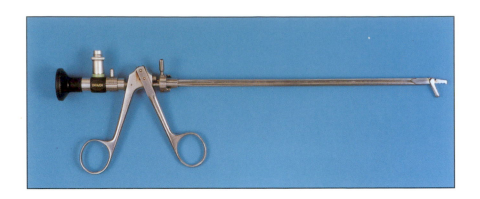

Figure 8.12
Storz stone-crushing forceps.

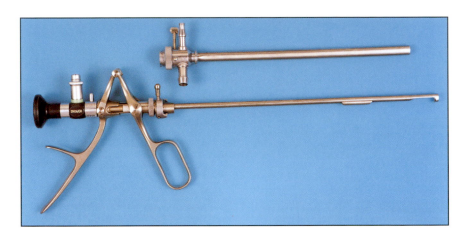

Figure 8.13
Mauermayer's stone punch.

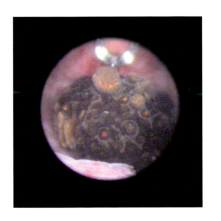

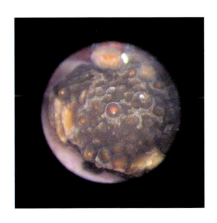

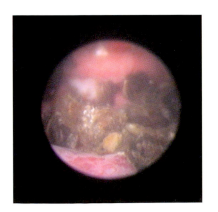

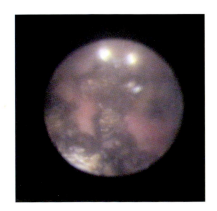

Figure 8.14
Crushing a small calculus with Mauermayer's stone punch.

Figure 8.15
Freyer's classical lithotrite.

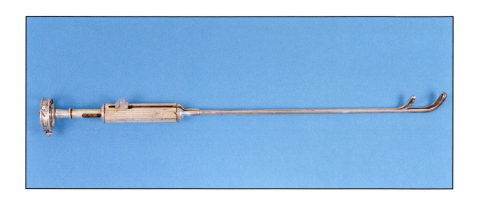

The classical blind lithotrite, however, (Fig. 8.15), remains the most effective and rapid instrument for all but the smallest stones and it is a pity that its use is a skill which seems to be dying out, despised by a generation of urologists reared on electrohydraulic or ultrasonic lithotriptors[10].

In classical litholapaxy the bladder should be about half-full. The lithotrite is well lubricated and passed with its blades closed. It is then opened and the female blade gently pressed down upon the trigone to form a hollow, into which the stone is allowed to roll (Fig. 8.16). The male blade is gently moved up and down until it gives the unmistakable sensation of feeling the stone in its jaws. Now the screw is locked and the instrument lifted up and moved each way to make sure that a fold of bladder mucosa has not been trapped in its jaws. Only then is the handle turned to crack the stone (Fig. 8.17).

The process is repeated as many times as is necessary to reduce the fragments to a size that will go down the resectoscope sheath. The instrument is then closed and removed. The resectoscope sheath is passed on its obturator and the fragments of stone are

Figure 8.16
Depress the bladder with the female blade until the stone rolls into its jaws.

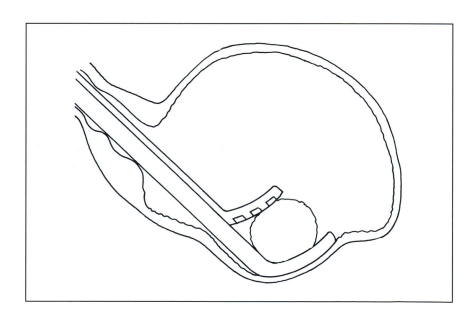

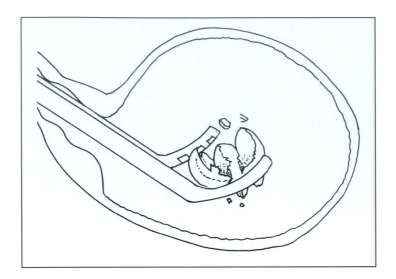

Figure 8.17
Once the stone is felt, lift it up to make sure the bladder has not been caught, and then crush it.

evacuated with the Ellik. The resectoscope telescope is passed to make sure that all the smallest bits have been removed. If any remain, they can often be eased out with the loop or crushed with the stone forceps.

When there has been a large stone which has been present for a long time it is prudent to take a mucosal biopsy of any suspicious area in view of the occasional complication of squamous cell cancer[11].

When the patient has a bulky middle lobe it can be difficult to see the stone. It is then more convenient to resect most of the middle lobe, then crush and evacuate the stone, and complete the transurethral resection in the usual way.

Diverticula of the bladder

Small saccules are commonly present in association with prostatic obstruction and can be disregarded (Fig. 8.18). Larger diverticula must always be fully examined by passing the cystoscope inside them to rule out cancer or a stone; be particularly suspicious of a diverticulum whose opening is oedematous or inflamed. If you cannot see inside clearly, make sure the diverticulum is innocent by means of a CT scan. When they harbour a stone or a tumour, or when there is continuing infection, the diverticulum should be removed, but since the prostate is often quite a small one, it is easier to perform the prostatectomy transurethrally and then go on to do the diverticulectomy in the usual way[12].

Figure 8.18
Multiple small diverticula often found with a trabeculated bladder.

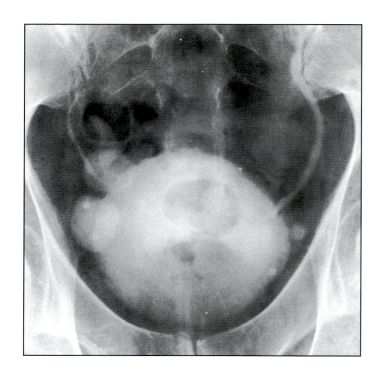

Urethral strictures and transurethral resection

Strictures may be found in patients who need transurethral resection of a bladder tumour. To allow the passage of the resectoscope it is necessary to dilate them or perform an optical urethrotomy. The optical urethrotome (Fig. 8.19) may be passed over a guide-wire or a

Figure 8.19
Sachse optical urethrotome (Storz).

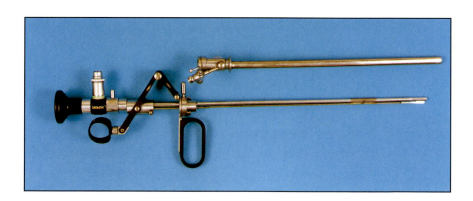

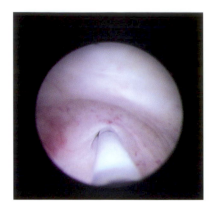

Figure 8.20
A guide wire or ureteric catheter may be passed through the stricture if the way through is not clear.

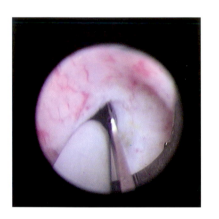

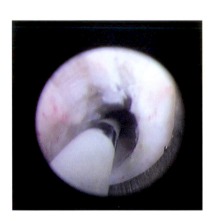

Figure 8.21
Internal optical urethrotomy using a ureteric catheter as guide.

ureteric catheter if the way through the stricture cannot be seen clearly (Fig. 8.20). The incision is made at 12 o'clock right through the fibrous stricture into healthy tissue (Fig. 8.21). Urethrotomy by itself does not produce a long-lasting cure, indeed its results are virtually indistinguishable from traditional dilatation[13], and so every patient must be followed up with intermittent dilatation or self-catheterization. When there is a bladder tumour to be resected prudence suggests that dilatation may be preferable in view of the possible implantation of cancer cells into the raw area in the urethra, although such cases must be exceedingly rare.

References

1. Weaver RP, Noble MJ, Weigel JW. Correlation of ultrasound guided and digitally directed biopsies of palpable prostatic abnormalities. *J Urol* 1991; **145**: 516.
2. Stamey TA. Making the most out of six systematic sextant biopsies. *Urology* 1995; **45**: 2.
3. Meacham RB, Scardino PT, Hoffman GS *et al.* The risk of distant metastases after transurethral resection of the prostate versus needle biopsy in patients with localized prostate cancer. *J Urol* 1989; **142**: 320.

4. Duncan W, Catton CN, Warde P *et al*. The influence of transurethral resection of prostate on prognosis of patients with adenocarcinoma of the prostate treated by radical radiotherapy. *Radiother Oncol* 1994; **31**: 41.
5. Hassler O. Calcifications in the prostate gland and adjacent tissues: a combined biophysical and histological study. *Path. Microbiol* 1968; **31**: 97.
6. Emmet JL. Transurethral removal of large prostatic calculi. *Proc Staff Meet Mayo Clin* 1941; **16**: 289.
7. Trapnell J, Roberts JBM. Prostatic abscess. *Br J Surg* 1970; **57**: 565.
8. Meares EM, Stamey TA. Bacteriological localization patterns in bacterial prostatitis and urethritis. *Invest Urol* 1968; **5**: 492.
9. Blandy JP, Fowler CG. Prostate — inflammation. In: *Urology* 2nd edn. Oxford: Blackwell Science, 1996; 375–79.
10. Swift-Joly J. *Stone and Calculous Disease of the Urinary Organs*. London: Heinemann, 1929.
11. Tannenbaum SI, Carson CC, Tatum A, Paulson DF. Squamous carcinoma of the urinary bladder. *Urology* 1983; **22**: 597.
12. Blandy JP. *Operative Urology* 2nd edn. Oxford: Blackwell Science, 1986: 123–25.
13. Steenkamp JW, Heyns CF, de Kock MLS. Dilatation versus internal urethrotomy as out-patient treatment for male urethral stricture—a prospective, randomized clinical trial. *Br J Urol* 1996; **77**: Suppl 2 (11).

Chapter 9

Routine postoperative care after transurethral resection

In the recovery room

From the operating table the patient goes to the recovery room where, in addition to monitoring the usual vital signs, the airway, and the intravenous drip (if there is one) the nursing team pay particular attention to the three-way catheter and its irrigating system (Fig. 9.1).

Many surgeons prefer to use a two-way catheter, and rely on the patient's own urine to keep the bladder irrigated. If necessary,

Figure 9.1

Recovery room: vital signs are monitored; the three-way irrigating system is kept running briskly, and nursing staff keep an eye on the suprapubic region. The penile swab used for tamponade is removed before the patient returns to the ward.

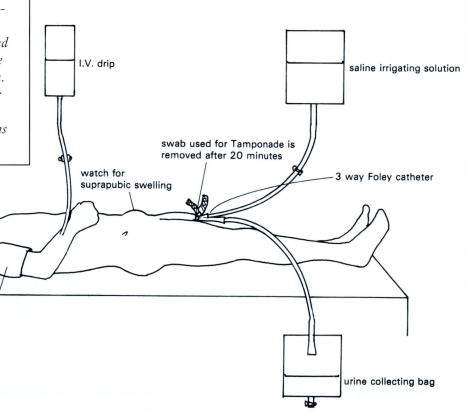

I.V. drip

saline irrigating solution

swab used for Tamponade is
removed after 20 minutes

watch for
suprapubic swelling

3 way Foley catheter

BP

urine collecting bag

intravenous fluids and a diuretic are given to encourage an adequate output of urine. The authors mistrust this system, fearing that it courts the risk of dilutional hyponatraemia, particularly in a patient with an inappropriate secretion of antidiuretic hormone, but it has many advocates.

Some surgeons prefer to leave the catheter to drain freely, only irrigating it with a hand-syringe if the flow is blocked. The disadvantage of this method is the risk of introducing infection whenever the bladder is irrigated with a syringe[1].

In the usual technique with the three-way catheter the purpose of the irrigation is to dilute the blood so that a clot will not form to block the catheter. The rate of inflow of the saline is adjusted from time to time to keep the outflow a pale pink *vin rosé* colour, and as a rule the rate of inflow can be cut down after about 20 minutes.

Blocked catheter

1. The bag may be too full and its valve squeezed shut (Fig. 9.2). For this reason the drainage bags should be emptied long before they are full.
2. A small clot may have obstructed the catheter.
3. A chip of prostate may have stuck in the eye of the catheter.

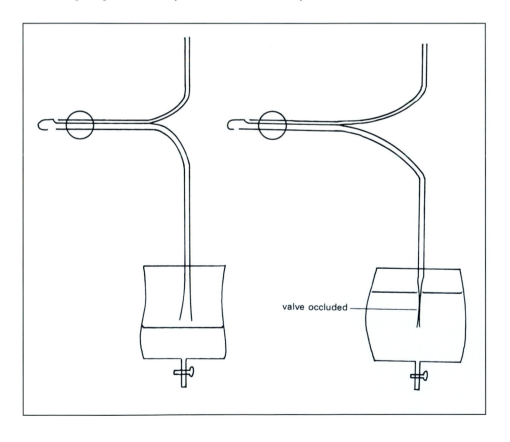

valve occluded

In both these latter cases the first thing is to apply a bladder syringe to the end of the catheter and give it a good suck: this will often start the flow. If not, some of the irrigant should be drawn up in the syringe until it is about half-full, and about 20 ml injected before smartly aspirating again with the object of clearing the eye of the catheter.

If neither of these tricks works, the catheter must be changed. It is no good persisting in vain attempts to syringe a catheter which is blocked: it will result in overdistension of the bladder which adds to the patient's distress and restlessness.

Let down the balloon of the catheter and withdraw it. Place a curved introducer in a new catheter and take care not to catch the bladder neck as you introduce it. More or less clear urine usually runs out at once, and when the bladder is empty irrigation can be started again.

If the bladder has been allowed to become full of clot then the patient should be returned to the theatre without delay. This is one of the chief advantages of having the recovery room close to the operating theatre: a message from the recovery room nurse will bring one of the surgical team within seconds, who can check the situation and make the decision to return the patient or not without delay. Experienced nursing staff usually know when it is time to return the patient and the young surgeon does well to take heed of their advice. It is far better to err on the side of caution than waste valuable time, while the patient may be continuing to bleed, fiddling with a bladder syringe and a hopelessly blocked catheter.

Figure 9.2
If the valved drainage bag is allowed to get too full, the valve is closed and drainage ceases.

Clot evacuation

Once reanaesthetized the patient is repositioned, cleaned and draped as for a transurethral resection. The catheter is removed and the resectoscope passed again. Often this will allow a clot or chip to emerge and the problem is solved, but it is always wise to look into the bladder and irrigate out any clots that may be there with the Ellik evacuator (Fig. 9.3). When the bladder has been emptied, check the cavity of the prostate for any source of bleeding. It is rare that you will find any: the bleeding (as with the tonsil bed) has usually stopped when the clot has been evacuated. Rarely you may find a little tag of prostate which seems to be keeping a small vein open: resect it and coagulate the vein.

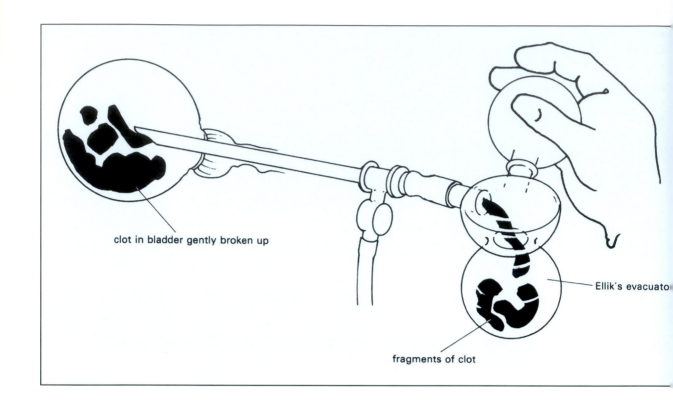

clot in bladder gently broken up

Ellik's evacuator

fragments of clot

Major reactionary haemorrhage

Mercifully very rare, major reactionary haemorrhage may take place without warning. If there is time, and the general condition of the patient permits, the bladder should be emptied with the Ellik and the source of bleeding coagulated, if possible, or controlled by traction on the Foley catheter. Exceptionally, the bleeding is impossible to control by these means, and it is necessary to open the patient and pack the prostate bed.

The retropubic space is opened through a Pfannenstiel incision. The bladder is retracted as for a Millin's prostatectomy and the capsule incised transversely[2]. All clot is evacuated and the prostatic bed firmly packed with gauze. Allow plenty of time for loss of blood to be restored, and then remove the pack, try to identify the source of bleeding, and suture the offending vessel. If the bleeding continues, pack it and close the wound with a large suprapubic tube in the bladder.

Fortunately this emergency is rare, but there are few urologists of experience who have not had to pack the prostate once or twice. The important thing is not to procrastinate when the patient is losing blood rapidly: it is better to have to explain an unexpected Pfannenstiel incision to a living patient than to his widow.

Figure 9.3
Clot retention. The resectoscope sheath is passed and the Ellik evacuator is used to break up the clot and suck it out.

Sedation

Transurethral resection is seldom painful unless the wall of the bladder or the trigone has been resected, or a large middle lobe has had to be removed. Then the patient may have an fierce desire to pass urine and the bladder may be thrown into involuntary detrusor spasms which nothing will control, and urine may escape alongside the catheter.

A sacral or caudal epidural anaesthetic minimizes this kind of postoperative discomfort and will last for several hours. Pethidine or morphine will relieve pain but do not prevent detrusor spasm, and they may lull the recovery staff into a sense of false security so that they may not realize that the pain and leakage are in fact due to a blocked catheter. Because transurethral resection is not usually a painful procedure, it is wise not to prescribe postoperative analgesic drugs as a routine in order to avoid this hazard. If the patient is in pain, find out why, before prescribing analgesia. Most commonly the patient who is apparently in pain will settle down as he regains full consciousness and can understand that there is a catheter in his penis.

Return to the ward

As soon as the patient has recovered consciousness and the irrigating system has settled down to an even flow, then the patient may go back to the ward. During the journey it is important that the irrigation is not inadvertently shut off, and as soon as the patient arrives on the ward the irrigating system should be checked to make sure that the fluid is running and that the bag has not become overfilled (Fig. 9.4). Thereafter the patient's vital signs are checked at intervals of 15, and later 30, minutes.

When the patient comes round he may well be hungry and thirsty and there is no reason why he should not be allowed to drink so long as he is not nauseated. Within 4 to 6 hours most patients are fully alert, may take a light meal, and start to drink as they please. If blood loss needs to be made up then the intravenous cannula should be retained until all the blood has been given. If the bleeding has stopped and the patient is taking fluids well there is no need to keep the drip up.

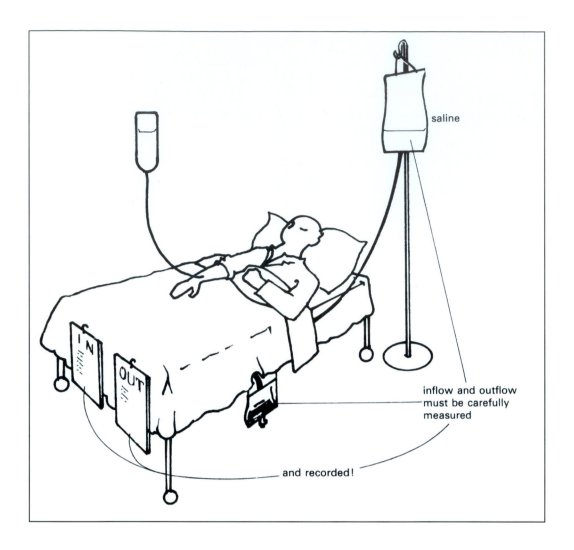

Recording the irrigating fluid

The volume of fluid run into the bladder and the urine collected should be continuously recorded and totted up every hour to make sure that there is no large discrepancy which might suggest that the bladder is becoming overdistended, or that there is an excessive loss of fluid into the veins (see page 47).

Ambulation

Patients should be encouraged to sit out of bed as soon as possible—the evening of their operation or the following morning—or as soon as the effects of the epidural anaesthetic have worn off. The next day they should be encouraged to walk around the ward carrying their catheter and the drip for the irrigating fluid if this is still needed (Fig. 9.5).

Figure 9.4
Return to the ward. Inflow and outflow must be measured. Ward staff should check that the penile swab has been removed. As the colour of the outflow becomes less blood-stained the rate of inflow is cut down.

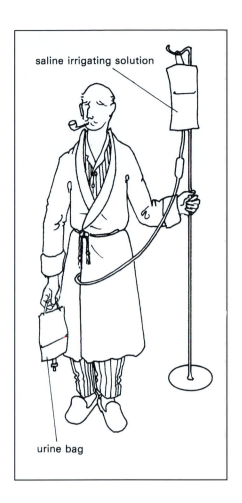

Irrigation

When the effluent is clear, or contains only a little staining of altered brownish blood, the irrigation may be discontinued—usually after about 12 hours.

Removing the catheter

Common sense dictates when the catheter should be removed. Sundays and public holidays are bad days to remove a catheter, and for the same reason it is better to remove the catheter early in the morning than late at night.

When a patient has had chronic retention with a huge floppy bladder year in and year out, it is unlikely that his detrusor will regain the ability to expel the urine for several days. Most patients, however, pass water within a few hours of removing the catheter.

If the catheter is taken out within 6–12 hours of the resection, as one may be tempted to do when the bleeding has been exceptionally well controlled, urine may escape from capsular perforations and give rise to stinging and pain on urination. For this reason it is usual to remove the catheter after about 48 hours. Warn the patient that removing the catheter is a little uncomfortable and ensure that it is taken out slowly and gently. The very apprehensive patient deserves a little sedation beforehand.

Failure to void after removing the catheter

There are three reasons for this:
1. The most common reason is that the patient finds it so uncomfortable to start to void that the process is inhibited. He shuts his external sphincter tightly and even when the bladder is painfully distended, cannot void.
2. The patient has detrusor failure from chronic retention.
3. Insufficient tissue may have been removed, usually at 2 or 10 o'clock, for when the prostatic capsule shrinks down a tiny lump becomes relatively large compared with the lumen of the prostatic urethra (Fig. 9.6).

When a patient cannot pass urine within an hour or two of removing the catheter one should not wait for the bladder to become painfully distended, but replace the catheter as soon as the patient has any discomfort, or whenever the bladder can be felt. Be aware of the pitfall of the patient with a big floppy detrusor who may be passing small amounts of urine but is quietly building up a huge residual.

Allow 3 or 4 days of rest, and then remove the catheter a second time and see if the patient can void. The man with the first, most common, type of failure to void will now do so without difficulty.

The patient with significant obstruction due to residual prostatic tissue should be returned to the theatre and the offending tissue resected: it is usually only a few grams.

Figure 9.5
First postoperative day. The patient may walk around, carrying his irrigating drip and urine bag.

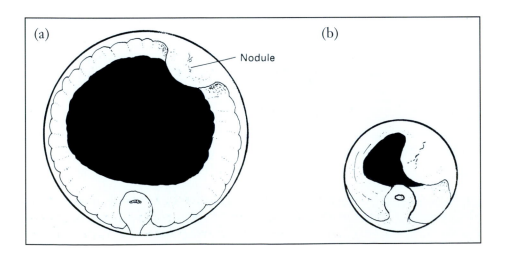

(a)   (b)   Nodule

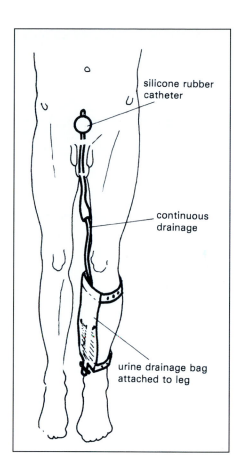

silicone rubber
catheter

continuous
drainage

urine drainage bag
attached to leg

Figure 9.6
If a small nodule of tissue has been left behind after removing a large prostate, leaving a large cavity, it is very easy to overlook it at the time (a), but it becomes all too obvious when the prostatic cavity has contracted (b).

The patient with detrusor failure poses a more serious problem. There is seldom any pain, but he soon returns to the state of chronic retention with overflow in which he arrived in hospital. In nearly every case the detrusor function returns after about 4 weeks of catheter drainage. He should be allowed to go home with an indwelling catheter on free drainage (Fig. 9.7). On no account should the patient be provided with a spigot or tap, or there will be a serious risk of accumulation of infected urine in the bladder with resulting septicaemia.

After about a month, the patient is readmitted to hospital overnight for the catheter to be removed, under antibiotic cover. The patient is carefully monitored to make sure that residual urine does not gradually accumulate: the best method is to check this with an ultrasound scan. Cholinergic drugs are often recommended for this type of detrusor failure but they do not work in practice when the problem is of long-standing.

Deliberate sphincterotomy

Some very old demented men with chronic retention have a detrusor which is irrevocably damaged and never recovers the strength to empty the bladder. A permanent indwelling catheter may not be tolerated, and may prevent them from being cared for in sheltered accommodation for the elderly. In such a patient it may be a kindness to perform an external sphincterotomy (see page 118) and fit him with a penile urinal, but such a decision will not be taken lightly and only in consultation with the geriatrician in overall charge of the care of the patient.

Going home

Most men can leave hospital after transurethral resection of the prostate or even a large bladder tumour within 4–5 days of the operation, but it is important to make sure that they understand that the raw area inside them will not be healed up completely for some time. They should rest quietly. Many patients (especially doctors, and practically all surgeons) think they can rush back to work simply because they have felt no pain. Nothing is more likely to give rise to secondary haemorrhage. Tell them they must take it easy. In reply to the inevitable question, 'What do you mean, Doctor?' a good guide is anything they would normally do in their carpet slippers (Fig. 9.8). They may potter around the house, go next door for a chat and have friends round to see them, but they must not play golf, walk the dog, dig the garden or mow the lawn. Surgeons must not operate. No one should drive a car.

This carpet-slipper convalescence should go on for 2 weeks after the patient has left hospital. It is designed to prevent the physical effort which might increase the pressure in the pelvic veins and provoke secondary haemorrhage.

After this time the patient should gradually return to normal life, increasing his activities day by day, go for walks, play a few holes of golf and go shopping. The rate of his progress will usually be regulated by the patient's frequency and urgency which take a little while to subside. Ideally this second period is one of getting back

Figure 9.7
If failure to resume voiding is due to atony of the detrusor, a period of continuous catheter drainage is necessary. The patient may go home wearing a silicone rubber catheter connected to a leg drainage bag. Never permit a spigot to be used.

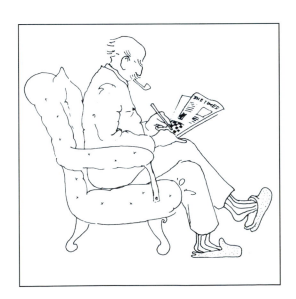

into training for a normal life, and if your patient can afford it, he should go away for a holiday in the sun before returning to work, or the equally strenuous life of modern-day retirement. The holiday should be postponed until 3 or 4 weeks after the operation, this being the risk period for secondary haemorrhage.

Fluid intake

During the period of carpet-slipper convalescence your patient should drink freely—about 3 l a day—so that the overconcentrated urine does not sting when he voids, and debris are washed away from the healing prostatic fossa. It matters not a jot what he drinks and there is no medical reason why he should not take a little alcohol if he wants to: one never encourages a patient to get drunk, but there is no physiological or pharmacological reason why he should be denied this little solace in time of trouble. After the first 2 weeks he may drink as much or as little fluid as he pleases.

Diet

There are no restrictions on what a man may or may not eat after transurethral surgery. Constipation is to be avoided since the passage of a stiff motion may provoke straining and start secondary haemorrhage. Plenty of bran and vegetables is sufficient for most men, and a bulk laxative for those inclined to be constipated, will keep postoperative bowel actions soft and comfortable.

Antibiotics

If prophylactic antibiotics have been given because the patient had been catheterized, or there was known urinary infection, there is no consensus as to how long they should be continued. It is probably wise to keep up the antibiotic cover until the catheter is removed, and for 24 hours thereafter. Where there is a special risk of systemic infection, e.g. in patients with implanted foreign bodies or mitral valve disease, a more prolonged course may be advisable and should be planned with the help of the patient's cardiologist and your microbiologist.

Figure 9.8
'Carpet-slipper' convalescence is enjoined for 2 weeks after leaving hospital.

References

1. Symes JM, Hardy DG, Sutherns K, Blandy JP. Factors reducing the rate of infection after transurethral surgery. *Br J Urol* 1972; **44**: 582.
2. Blandy JP. *Operative Urology* 2nd edn. Oxford: Blackwell Science, 1986: 168–76.
3. Hall JC, Christiansen KJ, England P *et al*. Antibiotic prophylaxis for patients undergoing transurethral resection of the prostate. *Urology* 1996; **47**: 852.
4. Emberton M, Neal DE, Black N *et al*. The National Prostatectomy Audit: the clinical management of patients during hospital admission. *Br J Urol* 1995; **75**: 301.

Chapter 10

Complications occurring during transurethral resection

Bleeding

Because bleeding is the chief cause of difficulty and danger in any form of prostatectomy, surgeons have been trying to discover how to limit blood loss for more than a century. The way to obtain haemostasis during the operation has been described (see page 68) and is usually sufficient to permit a clean resection for which no blood replacement is needed. Nevertheless from time to time haemorrhage can be copious, unexpected and daunting. However skilled the resector, it is always necessary to be prepared, to know the patient's haemoglobin and to have his blood grouped and serum saved in the laboratory. In very large prostates and very large bladder tumours where considerable blood loss is to be expected it is safer to have 2 units of blood standing by.

Adjuvant methods of limiting blood loss

Claims have been made that cooling the tissues with ice-cold irrigating fluid may reduce blood loss, but were based on resection of very small amounts of tissue. In theory, one would expect the natural clotting mechanisms to work best at normal temperature, and in practice the technique led to a sometimes alarming fall in core temperature[1–5]. Hypotensive anaesthesia was used extensively for retropubic prostatectomy some 30 years ago and is revived from time to time for transurethral surgery, but the benefit in terms of limiting blood loss must be offset by the risk of cerebrovascular accident and coronary thrombosis, both hazards of any surgical procedure in this age group.

Many other agents have been tried with the object of limiting blood loss, including oestrogens, injecting the prostate with vasoconstrictors, carbazochrome salicylate, kutapressin, oestrogens and aprotinin, all without significant benefit[6–10]. Cyclokapron and its precursor ε-amino-caproic acid were in vogue for a time, and then given up when it was found that they caused intraglomerular thrombosis[11-12]. They might have limited postoperative blood loss, but had no effect on bleeding during the operation. Dicynene, said to reduce capillary fragility, had no advantage when bleeding was serious[13].

More important than any of these adjuvant agents is a good technique of haemostasis at the time of operation, and to use a simple method of measuring blood loss in the operating theatre, e.g. a colorimeter to estimate the haemoglobin in the bucket[14].

Extraperitoneal perforation

This has been discussed above (see page 96). In practice danger only arises from perforations where large veins are opened and a large volume of fluid escapes into the circulation; it is rare for escape of fluid into the retropubic space to cause any trouble (Fig. 10.1(a)). However, occasionally fluid introduced with the Ellik evacuator does not suck back, or a change in the character of the respiration and a coldness and swelling of the suprapubic tissues may suggest that there has been a massive loss of fluid. As in most times in surgery when things go wrong they get worse if you dither and delay. Stop the resection. Have things made ready as soon as possible. Make a Pfannenstiel incision. Expose the bladder, open it between stay sutures and evacuate the clot. Complete the prostatectomy (if it is not already complete) by enucleating the remaining adenoma with the finger[15]. Get exact haemostasis by sutures, and if you can see the hole in the capsule, close it with a stitch. Only when all the bleeding is controlled should you close the wound with a suprapubic and urethral catheter and a drain to the retropubic space.

Intraperitoneal perforation

Small perforations into the perivesical tissues are not uncommon when resecting small tumours of the bladder and so long as you have secured good haemostasis and all the irrigating fluid is being recovered, no additional steps are required except that perhaps one should leave the catheter in for 4 rather than 2 days.

When the perforation has been made right through into the peritoneum (Fig. 10.1(b)) or, as is often the case, the perforation is obscured and accompanied by haemorrhage, then it is necessary to explore the abdomen. The bladder is again approached through a Pfannenstiel incision, opened between stay sutures, the clot evacuated, the bleeding controlled and the hole sewn up (Fig. 10.2). Then the peritoneum should be opened to note whether there is any blood-stained fluid inside. If there is, the adjacent loops of small and large bowel should be pulled out and searched for diathermy damage. A hole in the small bowel is closed in its transverse axis (Fig. 10.3). A hole in the colon should be protected with a temporary loop-colostomy.

Figure 10.1

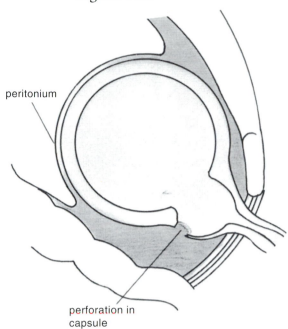

peritonium

perforation in
capsule

*(a) Extraperitoneal perforation; fluid extravasates
around the prostate and the base of the bladder.*

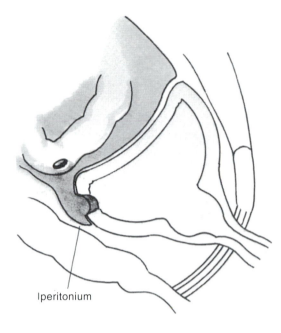

Iperitonium

*(b) Intraperitoneal perforation; the main
danger is of inadvertent injury to the bowel.*

Figure 10.2
*As soon as the bladder is
opened the perforation is
obvious.*

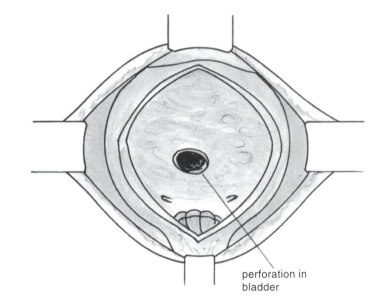

perforation in
bladder

Figure 10.3
*A small burn in the small
bowel is oversewn in its
transverse axis.*

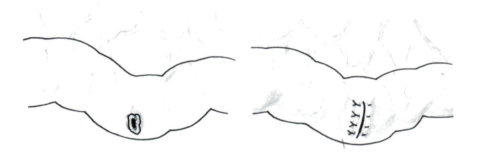

Perforation into the rectum

Although this is much dreaded, it is excessively rare. In one unit it was only seen once in >5000 resections, in a period when three such cases were referred from other centres following open operations, usually when the prostate was malignant. In the first instance a catheter should be passed and left *in situ* for about 3 weeks, during which time the patient is carefully observed.

The main danger is faeces entering the bladder and causing severe infection. If this occurs, a defunctioning colostomy and a suprapubic cystostomy should be set up without delay. After about 6 weeks most of these fistulae will have healed, and in the rare case that persists the fistula can be closed through a perineal approach or by one of Parks' operations using a sleeve of rectal wall[16,17].

Broken sheath

In days when sheaths were generally made of plastic they sometimes broke across, leaving the tip in the urethra. Even today the tip of a steel sheath may come away. Occasionally one can see the edge of the detached portion with a cystoscope and draw it out with biopsy forceps (Fig. 10.4). An alternative trick is to pass a Foley catheter through the lumen of the detached portion, leave it for 10 to14 days, and when the catheter is removed the piece of sheath will usually come away (Fig. 10.5).

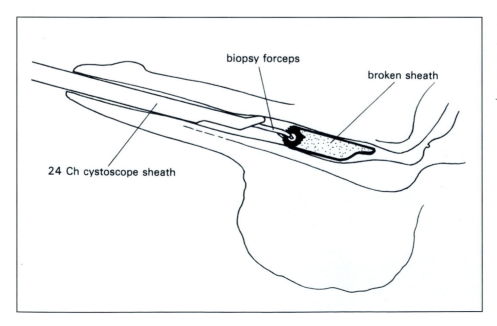

biopsy forceps

broken sheath

24 Ch cystoscope sheath

Figure 10.4
A broken-off tip of a resectoscope may be recovered with a biopsy forceps.

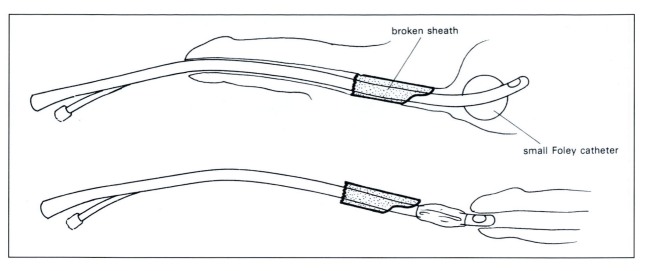

broken sheath

small Foley catheter

Figure 10.5
If a small Foley catheter can be passed through the broken fragment of resectoscope sheath, it is left for about 10 days; when it is removed, the sheath comes with it.

Broken loop

A fragment of inert wire broken off in the course of a transurethral resection can do no possible harm unless in the fullness of time it migrates into the bladder and acts as a nucleus for a stone to form. By all means look for it and remove it with a biopsy forceps if you find it, but otherwise, complete the resection with another loop. An X-ray in the postoperative period will reveal the loop (Fig. 10.6), but if the patient is comfortable there is no need to hunt for it. What you tell the patient is of course for you to decide in the interests of the peace of mind of your patient rather than what you fear his lawyers might say, but you will probably find that it simplifies things to tell him, explaining that there are many old soldiers who still carry with them bullets and shrapnel fragments from past wars, and many surgeons routinely use metal clips for haemostasis. A man may well feel aggrieved and insulted if he finds out later and you had not told him.

Figure 10.6
Plain X-ray showing resectoscope loop in the prostate. It caused no trouble and was left alone.

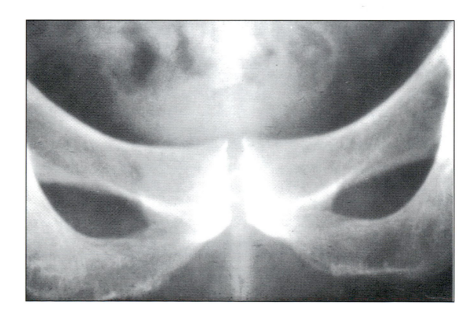

Explosions

The mixture of hydrogen and oxygen formed by hydrolysis of water by diathermy sparks, along with air introduced in the irrigating fluid, collects into a bubble at the vault of the bladder. This is sometimes an explosive mixture, so if you are resecting tumour from the vault, push down on the suprapubic region to indent the vault and displace the bubble away from the loop. The writers have never seen this terrible complication but the accounts of it in the literature make grim reading[18].

Obturator jump

If a bladder tumour is situated on the lateral wall of the bladder, resection may be complicated by brisk spasms of the adductors of the ipsilateral leg—the obturator jump. This occurs when low frequency harmonic currents generated by the diathermy stimulate the obturator nerve. Apart from giving you a box on the ears, this surprising event may cause you to perforate the wall of the bladder with the cutting loop. There is no certain way to avoid this phenomenon, but steps can be taken to reduce the likelihood of it taking place.

First, be aware of the possibility whenever you are resecting tumours near the ureteric orifice.

Turn down the current until it is barely cutting. The obturator nerve may no longer be stimulated. Next, ask your anaesthetist to intubate the patient and paralyse his muscles. Curare-related agents work by blocking depolarizatrion of the neuromuscular end plates, but this blockade can be overcome by supramaximal nerve stimulation. Theoretically paralysis with agents such as suxamethonium, which depolarize the end plates and prevent repolarization, ought to overcome the problem, but their action is short-lived, and repeated administration may lead to other problems so that anaesthetists are understandably not enthusiastic to use repeated doses.

The obturator nerve may be anaesthetized locally by injecting local anaesthetic directly into the nerve (Fig. 10.7). Using a long spinal needle aim for the obturator foramen, entering the needle halfway between the mid-inguinal point and the pubic tubercle, aiming downwards and medially, aspirating and injecting alternately until the bony medial edge of the obturator foramen is encountered. If the femoral vein is inadvertently entered, press on the puncture for 5 minutes.

Figure 10.7
Injection of local anaesthetic into the obturator nerve.

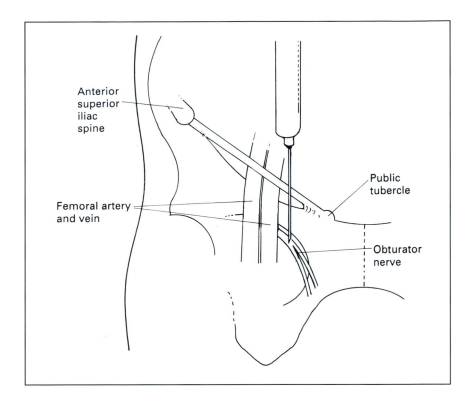

Erection

Penile erection can develop insidiously and the operator must constantly be on the lookout for it, for it is exceedingly dangerous. It is the authors' experience that erection is most common in patients too lightly anaesthetized, often by an inexperienced anaesthetist.

The first sign that anything is going wrong may be that the resectoscope seems to be unduly tight in the urethra, or that the view has become obscured by new bleeding. Feel the penis; early engorgement is quite obvious. Stop now, before it is too late.

Fortunately it is now quite easy to reverse the erection with an injection directly into the corpus cavernosum of metaraminol or phenylepinephrine (1 mgm) diluted in normal saline. Hypotensive drugs may be needed, e.g. phentolamine[19]. The erection subsides immediately and the operation can be continued.

Failure to recognise that an erection is taking place and failure to reverse it may result in the resectoscope being forced out of the urethra, with the result that the operator may easily mistake the external sphincter for prostate, and resect it. The result is irreversible incontinence (Fig. 10.8).

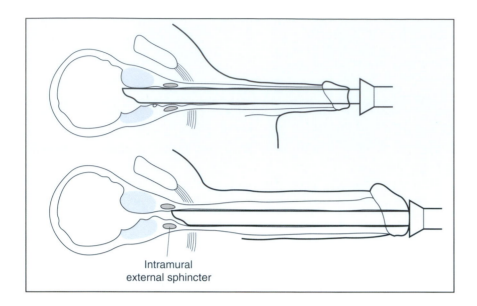

Intramural
external sphincter

Figure 10.8
During an erection the short flaccid penis becomes elongated, forcing the resectoscope out. It is easy to mistake external sphincter for prostate, especially when bleeding confuses your view.

The 1 hour rule and transurethral resection

An interesting myth has been handed down from one generation of resectors to the next, without any basis in measurement or experiment, namely that resection must be completed within 60 minutes or disaster will befall. The myth probably took its origin in the early days of transurethral resection when the surgeon often gave his own spinal anaesthetic, and patients began to recover sensation after about an hour.

Clearly, the longer the operation goes on, the more time there is for blood to be lost and irrigating fluid to enter the veins, and if the resection takes more than 1 hour, it usually means that the gland is very large (when there is more likely to be more of both) or the resector has been unduly slow in removing what gland there is. Time alone is no more relevant to endoscopic than to any other kind of surgery, and if you can make a better job of the operation by taking 61 minutes it is illogical to call a halt at 59.

While the 1 hour rule is certainly great nonsense there is never any excuse for dawdling. This is nothing new in surgery; operating time is not wasted by taking care and trouble over the steps of any operation, but in indecision—fiddling about and wondering what to do next. It is a commonplace in surgery that master craftsmen neither hurry nor watch the clock, but they never waste a movement. So it should be in transurethral resection. Keep your landmarks ever in view; know where you are and what you are cutting. Cut with a confident rhythm and stop the bleeding as you go. Transurethral resection is no work for the picker and scratcher.

The TUR syndrome

Early in the history of transurethral resection it was recognized that if distilled water was allowed to run into the circulation it would lead to haemolysis, haemoglobinuria and possibly even renal failure[20-23] (Fig. 10.9). Accordingly a number of non-ionizing solutions were introduced which would be more or less isotonic and fail to cause haemolysis, e.g. 2.5% glucose, Cytal—a proprietary mixture of sorbitol and mannitol, and 1.5% glycine.

Although these solutions avoided the risk of haemolysis, they did not avoid the dangers that arose from intravenous infusion of a large volume of water into the blood. This dilutes the normal electrolytes,

Figure 10.9
The hazards of using distilled water as the irrigating medium.

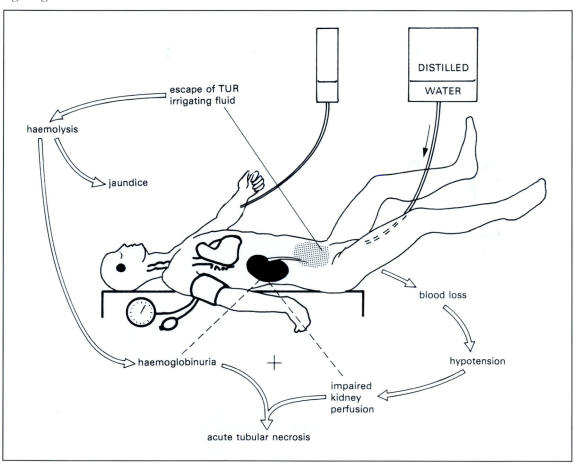

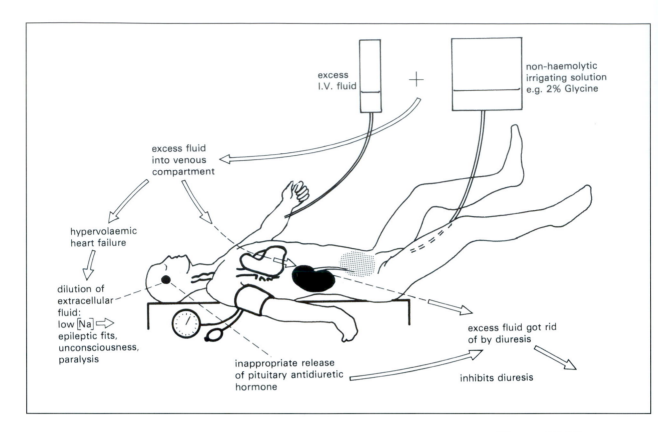

excess
I.V. fluid

non-haemolytic
irrigating solution
e.g. 2% Glycine

excess fluid
into venous
compartment

hypervolaemic
heart failure

dilution of
extracellular
fluid:
low [Na] ⇨
epileptic fits,
unconsciousness,
paralysis

inappropriate release
of pituitary antidiuretic
hormone

excess fluid got rid
of by diuresis

inhibits diuresis

Figure 10.10
The dilutional syndrome.

especially sodium leading to a lowering of the membrane potential on the cell wall which is necessary for nerve conduction and muscle contraction. This is soon followed by an increase in intracellular water, resulting in cell oedema (Fig. 10.10).

A normal patient can cope with a suprisingly large volume of water added to his bloodstream in this way, responding with a prompt diuresis that gets rid of the surplus water. But not all transurethral resection patients are normal; many are already on the brink of heart failure, and in as many as 25% there is an inappropriate secretion of pituitary antidiuretic hormone[24]. An additional factor, hitherto unnoticed, may be the effect of endotoxins due to bacteraemia during the resection[25].

It is possible to measure the quantity of fluid escaping into the patient if a special weighing machine is added to the ordinary operating table[26]. Nowadays it is also possible to monitor the concentration of sodium in the blood with a sodium-sensing electrode[27], or more easily, by adding a little alcohol to the irrigating fluid and constantly monitoring the expired air with a breathalyser[28].

Many techniques have been used to avoid the TUR syndrome. A suprapubic cannula and the continuous irrigating cystoscope of Iglesias are commonly used[29]. In practice the TUR syndrome is rarely seen in most modern departments, partly because of these precautions, and perhaps because of sparing use of intravenous fluids[30,31] and careful measurement of the volumes of fluid that are irrigated in and out of the bladder.

Diagnosis

The diagnosis of the TUR syndrome calls for a high degree of awareness on the part of the urological team. It may be ushered in with restlessness and hypertension, and rapidly proceed to what appears to be a *grand mal* seizure. Transient blindness is sometimes seen.

Treatment

In a patient who is not too ill, and is having a good diuresis, it is safe to wait and let him get better. However when there are epileptiform seizures, signifying cerebral oedema, it is safer to give 50 ml of 29.2% saline. This is done slowly, through a central venous cannula[32] because it is not without its own risks of causing further cerebral damage[33].

Glycine as an irrigant has come in for some criticism because in theory it may lead to an accumulation of ammonia[34] and oxalate[35].

References

1. Madsen PO, Kaveggia L, Atassi SA. The effect of oestrogens (premarin) and regional hypothermia on blood loss during transurethral prostatectomy. *J Urol* 1964; **92**: 314.
2. Madsen PO, Bohlman DC, Madsen RE. Local hypothermia during transurethral surgery. *Anesthesia Analges* 1965; **44**: 734.
3. Robson CT, Sales JL. Effect of local hypothermia on blood loss during transurethral resection of the prostate. *J Urol* 1966; **95**: 393.
4. Serrao A, Mallik MK, Jones PA, Hendry WF, Wickham JEA. Hypothermic prostatic resection. *Br J Urol* 1976; **48**: 685.
5. Walton JK, Rawstron RE. The effect of local hypothermia on blood loss during transurethral resection of the prostate. *Br J Urol* 1981; **53**: 258.
6. Creevy CD. Aids to hemostasis during transurethral prostatic resection. *J Urol* 1965; **93**: 80.
7. Madsen PO, Straugh AE, Barquin OP, Malek GH. The lack of hemostatic effect of polyestradiolphosphate and carbazochrome salicylate in transurethral prostatectomy. *J Urol* 1968; **99**: 786.
8. Weisenthal CL, Meade RC, Owenby J, Irwin RI. An investigation of kutapressin as a hemostatic agent in transurethral surgery of the prostate. *J Urol* 1961; **86**: 346.
9. Pearson BS. The effects of Trasylol and aminocaproic acid in post prostatectomy haemorrhage. *Br J Urol* 1969; **41**: 602.
10. Lawrence ACK, Ward-McQuaid JN, Holdom GL. Effect of EACA on blood loss after retropubic prostatectomy. *Br J Urol* 1966; **38**: 308.
11. Madsen PO, Strauch AE. The effect of aminocaproic acid on bleeding following transurethral prostatectomy. *J Urol* 1996; **96**: 255.
12. Vinnicombe J, Shuttleworth KED. Aminocaproic acid in the control of haemorrhage after prostatectomy. *Lancet* 1966; **1**: 230.
13. Symes JM, Offen DN, Lyttle JA, Blandy JP, Chaput de Saintonge DM. The effect of Dicynene on blood loss during and after transurethral resection of the prostate. *Br J Urol* 1975; **47**: 203.
14. Wilson RG, Smith D, Paton G, Gollock JM, Bremner DN. Prophylactic subcutaneous heparin does not increase operative blood loss during and after transurethral resection of the prostate. *Br J Urol* 1988; **62**: 246.
15. Blandy JP. *Operative Urology* 2nd edn. Oxford: Blackwell Science, 1986: 400–3.
16. Tiptaft RC, Motson RW, Costello AJ, Paris AMI, Blandy JP. Fistulae involving rectum and urethra: the place of Parks' operations. *Br J Urol* 1983; **55**: 711.
17. Blandy JP. *Operative Urology* 2nd edn. Oxford: Blackwell Science, 1986; 357–59.
18. Hansen RE, Iversen P. Bladder explosions during uninterrupted transurethral resection of the prostate. *Scan J Urol Nephrol* 1979; **13**: 211.

19. McNicholas TA, Thomson K, Rogers HS, Blandy JP. The pharmacological management of erections during transurethral surgery. *Br J Urol* 1987; **64**: 435.
20. Creevy CD. Hemolytic reactions during transurethral prostatic resection. *J Urol* 1947; **58**: 125.
21. Bunge RG, Barker AP. Hemolysis during transurethral prostatic resection. *J Urol* 1948; **60**: 122.
22. Creevy CD, Reiser MP. The importance of hemolysis in transurethral prostatic resection: severe and fatal reactions associated with the use of distilled water *J Urol* 1963; **89**: 900.
23. Beirne GJ, Madsen PO, Burns RO. Serum electrolyte and osmolarity changes following transurethral resection of the prostate. *J Urol* 1954; **93**: 83.
24. Rao PN. Fluid absorption during urological endoscopy. *Br J Urol* 1987; **60**: 93.
25. Sohn MH, Vogt C, Heinen G, Erkens M, Nordmeyer N, Jakse G. Fluid absorption and circulating endotoxins during transurethral resection of the prostate. *Br J Urol* 1993; **72**: 605.
26. Coppinger SW, Lewis CA, Milroy EJG. A method of measuring fluid balance during transurethral resection of the prostate. *Br J Urol* 1995; **76**: 66.
27. Watkins-Pitchford JM, Payne SR, Rennie CD, Riddle PR. Hyponatraemia during transurethral resection: its practical prevention. *Br J Urol* 1984; **56**: 676.
28. Hahn RG. Ethanol monitoring of extravascular absorption of irrigating fluid. *Br J Urol* 1993; **72**: 766.
29. Iglesias JJ, Stams UK. How to prevent the TUR syndrome. *Urologe* 1975; **14**: 287
30. Gale DW, Notley RG. TURP without TURP syndrome. *Br J Urol* 1985; **57**: 708.
31. Goel CM, Badenoch DF, Fowler CG, Blandy JP, Tiptaft RC. Transurethral resection syndrome: a prospective study. *Eur Urol* 1992; **21**: 15.
32. Worthley LIG, Thomas PD. Treatment of hyponatraemic seizures with intravenous 29.2% saline. *Br Med J* 1986; **292**: 168.
33. Arieff AI. Management of hyponatraemia. *Br Med J* 1993; **307**: 305.
34. Shepard RL, Kraus SE, Babayan RK, Siroky MB. The role of ammonia toxicity in the post transurethral prostatectomy syndrome. *Br J Urol* 1987; **60**: 349.
35. Fitzpatrick JM, Kassidass GP, Rose GA. Hyperoxaluria following glycine irrigation for transurethral prostatectomy. *Br J Urol* 1981; **53**: 250.

Chapter 11

Late complications of transurethral resection

Infective complications

Septicaemic shock

Different incidences of bacteraemia are reported after transurethral resection ranging from as low as 1.6% to 58%, more commonly when the urine is infected before operation[1-3]. Disturbingly, as many as 55% of men were found to have positive blood cultures even though their preoperative urine had been sterile[4], while if bacterial endotoxins were measured the proportion rose even higher[5]. Fortunately only a small proportion of men in whom bacteria or endotoxins are found go on to develop septicaemic shock, which is relatively rare and always unexpected. Septicaemic shock is most likely to occur on the day of operation, or when the catheter is removed.

The warning is given by the development of restlessness, a high fever and rigors. At first the patient is flushed and it is at this stage that urgent action is necessary. Blood is taken for microbiological culture and through the same needle a large dose of the appropriate bactericidal antibiotic is given, taking advice from the hospital laboratory who will know which organism is most probably responsible. This is followed by intravenous fluid, and as soon as possible, a central venous catheter is inserted to monitor the pressure in the right atrium (Fig. 11.1).

From now on the patient is monitored very closely, preferably in the Intensive Care Unit where the rapid changes which take place with overperfusion or underperfusion can be monitored and corrected. Fortunately death from septicaemic shock after transurethral resection is now rare, although it is still dangerous in men over 80[6-7].

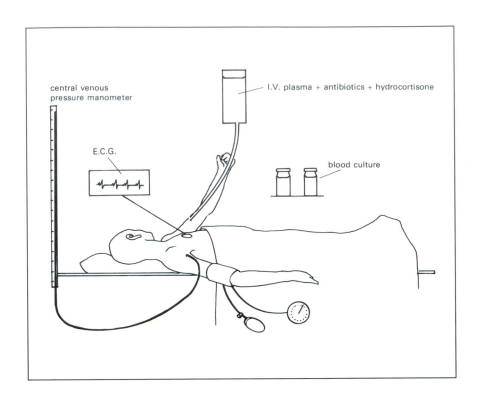

Figure 11.1
Septicaemic shock: the essentials of management.

central venous pressure manometer

I.V. plasma + antibiotics + hydrocortisone

E.C.G.

blood culture

Urinary infection

The reported incidence of urinary infection after transurethral resection varies from 6 to 100%. Much can be done to reduce infection by strict attention to aseptic drill when changing the catheter bag and when irrigating the bladder. If organisms enter the closed system it becomes a culture for organisms which are rapidly carried up into the bladder on the interface of bubbles[8]. Experience and quality control over the management of the catheter is one major reason for bringing urological patients together in one ward area. Even so, the incidence of urinary infection inexorably rises when any catheter has been in the bladder for more than 5 days, by which time a continuous biofilm of bacteria has come to coat the catheter from external meatus to bladder.

Fortunately the clinical effects of this bacterial colonization of the bladder are seldom of any consequence. Upper tract infection, as judged by rigors, a high temperature, or pain in the loin, is rare. Bacteraemia (as pointed out above) is even more rare. As a rule, within a few days of removing the catheter, the infected system has cleansed itself and infection which persists for more than 6 weeks after transurethral resection is so unusual that it makes one suspect persistent residual urine or a diverticulum.

Epididymitis

Once the bane of open prostatectomy, epididymitis is so rarely seen in hospital that the old practice of routine prophylactic vasectomy has long been given up. However its true incidence has probably been underestimated, and in the National Prostatectomy Study it occurred in 5% of men after they had left hospital[9]. When epididymitis does occur it may give rise to systemic illness out of proportion to the local signs, and require intensive antibiotic treatment, strict rest in bed, and elevation of the scrotum. If unchecked, epididymitis may proceed to suppuration and even loss of a testicle.

Urethritis

The catheter always provokes some discharge of mucus around the catheter. The normal secretions of the urethra accumulate at the external meatus to form a crust which should be cleansed regularly to remove a potential source of infection. In some patients there is an unusually severe reaction to the catheter, and may be followed by a stricture, probably from chemical or allergic irritation[10,11].

Osteomyelitis

One very rare infective complication of transurethral resection is vertebral osteomyelitis which is presumably a late aftermath of bacteraemia although patients who develop this have seldom had any noteworthy postoperative symptoms (Fig. 11.2). The infection begins in the intervertebral disk, and typically the patient complains of backache which comes on several weeks or months after the operation, is difficult to localize and steadily gets worse. There are almost no physical signs, and it is only when eventually the characteristic erosion of the vertebral body is demonstrated by Computerized Tomography or Magnetic Resonance Imaging that the diagnosis is made. Intensive treatment with antibiotics usually cures the condition quickly. The difficulty is to make the diagnosis.

Figure 11.2
X-ray showing osteomyelitis of vertebra.

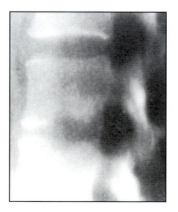

Deep venous thrombosis and pulmonary embolism

Clinically detectable deep vein thrombosis is rarely found[9,12,13] unless deliberately sought with labelled human serum albumen, but there is no room for complacency. Pulmonary embolism was diagnosed in 11 out of the 166 questionnaires analysed by the National Confidential Enquiry into Perioperative Deaths in 1993/1994, although the true proportion might well have been somewhat higher[14]. There is no consensus as to what precautions ought to be taken (see page 61), and somewhat disturbingly, 7 out of the 11 deaths reported to NCEPOD were given some type of anti-thromboembolism prophylaxis. There is a fertile field here for future research.

Cerebrovascular accident

From time to time an elderly man with a cardiac history or a previous small stroke comes into hospital, undergoes a transurethral resection, does well, and returns rejoicing to his family. A few weeks later he dies with a sudden stroke and the urologist blames himself feeling that perhaps if no operation had been done the patient might have survived. It appears that there is however no increased risk, unless the patient has had a history of cerebral or myocardial infarction[15] within the last 3 months.

Much concern has been raised recently following retrospective epidemiological studies which compared the long-term aftermath of open with transurethral prostatectomy. This came to the disturbing conclusion that men who underwent transurethral resection developed more cardiovascular illness in later life than those who underwent open surgery[16,17]. The cases had been operated on many years previously when transurethral surgery was offered only to the less fit patients by a generation of surgeons who were more adept at open surgery. Subsequent studies have failed to confirm this finding[18,19] but the very suggestion has led to the setting up of a multi-centre prospective study in North America (which has not passed uncriticized[20,21]). The controversy has also engendered several studies which have looked at a possible relationship between transurethral surgery and later cardiovascular disease, as to which the evidence is at present conflicting[22–25]. These unexpected arguments have also lent added emphasis to the quest for alternatives to transurethral resection.

Secondary haemorrhage

Bleeding in the early postoperative phase has been dealt with on page 130. Very commonly there is a small secondary bleed about the 10th postoperative day (see page 137) which the patient should be warned about. In the National Prostatectomy Study it caused difficulty in passing urine in 10% of patients[9].

What is far less common is for haemorrhage to occur months or years later. Often there is some new cause for it, e.g. cancer of the bladder or kidney, and all cases require a complete urological investigation. But in a number of men all that can be found is some regrowth of the prostatic adenoma and after a biopsy to rule out cancer of the prostate, nothing else needs to be done. However, within this group is a small number who continue to bleed. For them it has been our experience that a further prostatectomy, perhaps retropubic, is the only way to effect a permanent cure.

Stricture

The true incidence of stricture after transurethral surgery is probably rather higher than is admitted in most series, and it depends on how the diagnosis is made[25]. If the patient has no symptoms he is unlikely to have his flow-rate measured, let alone his urethra investigated by urethrogram, urethroscopy, or urethral ultrasound. The usual problem is a narrowing just inside the external meatus, presenting about 8 weeks after the operation with the symptom of spraying on micturition. It is easily treated by regular dilatation using a short straight bougie which the patient can be taught to pass on himself. The annual toll of these strictures is diminishing thanks probably to the increasing use of narrow resectoscope sheaths and the use of prophylactic internal urethrotomy[26].

Other sites for postoperative stricture are at the penoscrotal junction, the bulb and the external sphincter (Fig. 11.3). Occasionally optical urethrotomy is required, but usually these strictures are easily managed by dilatation supplemented by regular self catheterization.

Figure 11.3
Main sites of post transurethral resection strictures.

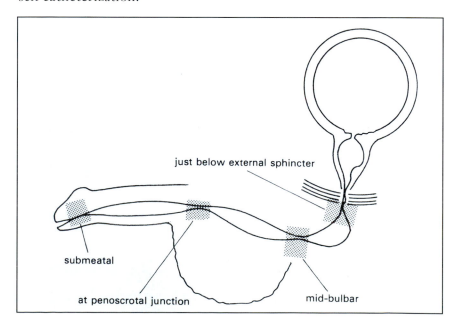

just below external sphincter

submeatal

at penoscrotal junction

mid-bulbar

Bladder neck stenosis

Formerly common after open prostatectomy this is rare after transurethral surgery. At an interval of some months after transurethral resection the patient comes back with a return of symptoms and is found to have a tight membrane at the level of the bladder neck (Fig. 11.4). It is easily put right with a urethrotome or a bee-sting electrode (Fig. 11.5), but it does tend to recur, perhaps because (as histology often shows) there is evidence of granuloma in the tissue. Bladder neck stenosis is not prevented by incision of the bladder neck[27].

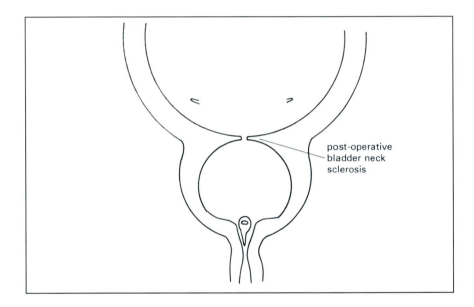

Figure 11.4
Bladder neck stenosis following prostatectomy.

Figure 11.5
Bladder neck stenosis. (a) The hole in the diaphragm is incised with the bee-sting electrode or Collings knife and then (b) the scar tissue is cut away all round.

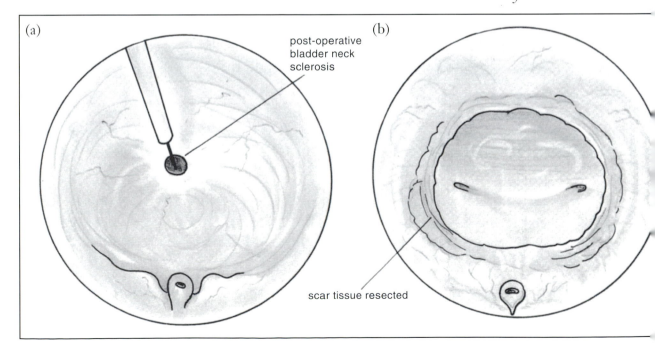

The need to repeat transurethral resection

One of the old criticisms of transurethral resection was that it was less thorough than surgical enucleation, and this was certainly true in the days when instrumentation was so poor. Today it is probably less common, but it was disturbing to find that in one large audit about 12% of transurethral resections were revision procedures[28]. Whether such regrowth is more common after transurethral than open prostatectomy is the object of a number of ongoing trials.

Incontinence

Far from causing incontinence, TUR often cures the incontinence which is present in a quarter of patients before operation; nevertheless one in 10 remain incontinent afterwards and the operation seems to cause incontinence in as many as 6%[9]; nothing is a greater disaster for an otherwise fit patient. In a proportion of cases the cause is poor selection of the patient whose symptoms were really due to detrusor instability from some other cause (see page 52). In such patients transurethral resection may change a picture of severe frequency into one of disabling incontinence.

Technical error at the time of operation can also cause incontinence. In such a patient endoscopy will show a tell-tale defect in the supramembranous external sphincter, usually at 10 or 2 o'clock, and perusal of the notes will yield the story that during the operation the patient developed an erection, the surgeon lost his way, and the sphincter was cut in mistake for adenoma (see page 145).

The investigation of post TUR incontinence requires uro-dynamic investigations to determine the state of the detrusor, and endoscopy to reveal the sphincter. The treatment is unsatisfactory: the choice is between wearing an incontinence appliance, a Cunningham clip, and having an artificial sphincter implanted. The problem with the Cunningham clip and the artificial sphincter is that the pressure needed to keep the urine in may be greater than that of the blood in the pelvic veins, so that ischaemic necrosis of the urethra may develop at the site of wearing the clip, or around the balloon of the Brantley Scott device[28,29].

Sexual dysfunction after transurethral resection

Recent studies have identified three separate elements to sexual dissatisfaction after transurethral surgery. The first is retrograde ejaculation, about which urologists have been aware for many years, and should routinely warn their patients since it occurs in about two out of three men[9]. It is probably caused by the removal of the bladder neck which normally closes during ejaculation, and is necessarily removed along with the obstructing adenoma.

The second component is erectile impotence. For many years this was given little thought, but some 70% of men are still sexually active in their 70s, and of these 10% to 30% will be rendered impotent afterwards[9,31–33].

There is a third component, namely the lack of the sensation of orgasm. This may relate to a deficiency in contraction of muscular tissue in the prostate and seminal vesicles. At any event some patients experience this after transurethral resection, although relatively few complain of it.

For the surgeon the crucial thing is that these matters are discussed with the patient before the operation, particularly when there is no life-threatening complication such as ureteric obstruction or severe infection, and especially in the younger patient who may not have completed his family. It was disturbing to find in one large audit that a note had been made to the effect that these matters had been discussed with the patient at the time of getting consent in less than 30% of records[34].

References

1. Kiely EA, McCormack T, Cafferkey MT, Faliner FR, Butler MR. Study of appropriate antibiotic therapy in transurethral prostatectomy. *Br J Urol* 1989; **64**: 61.
2. Hall JC, Christiansen KJ, England P *et al*. Antibiotic prophylaxis for patients undergoing transurethral resection of the prostate. *Urology* 1996; **47**: 852.
3. Ibrahim AIA, Bilal NE, Shetty SD, Patil KP, Gomaa H. The source of organisms in the post-prostatectomy bacteremia of patients with pre-operative sterile urine. *Br J Urol* 1993; **72**: 770.
4. Robinson MRG, Arudpragasam ST, Sahgal SM *et al*. Bacteraemia resulting from prostatic surgery: the source of bacteria. *Br J Urol* 1982; **37**: 551.
5. Sohn MH, Vogt C, Heinen G *et al*. Fluid absorption and circulating endotoxins during transurethral resection of the prostate. *Br J Urol* 1993; **72**: 605.
6. Phair JP. Approach to bacteremia (Gram positive/negative and septic shock). In: Kelley WN (ed.) *Textbook of Internal Medicine*. Philadelphia: Lippincott, 1989: 1796–1800.
7. Edwards JD. Management of septic shock. *Br Med J* 1993; **306**: 1661.
8. Ramsay JWA, Garnham AJ, Mulhall AB *et al*. Biofilms, bacteria and bladder catheters. *Br J Urol* 1989; **64**: 395.
9. Neal DE. The National Prostatectomy Audit. *Br J Urol* 1997; **79**: Suppl 2, 69.
10. Bailey MJ, Shearer RJ. The role of internal urethrotomy in the prevention of urethral stricture following transurethral resection of prostate. *Br J Urol* 1985; **57**: 81.
11. Blandy JP. Urethral stricture. *Postgrad Med J* 1980; **56**: 383.
12. Hedlund PO. Post-operative venous thrombosis in benign prostatic disease: a study of 316 patients using the ^{125}I fibrinogen uptake test. *Scand J Urol Nephrol* 1976; Suppl 27.
13. Parr NJ, Lohn CS, Desmond AD. Transurethral resection of the prostate without withdrawal of Warfarin therapy. *Br J Urol* 1989; **64**: 632.
14. Lunn JN, Devlin HB, Hoile RW. *The Report of the National Confidential Enquiry into Perioperative Deaths 1993/1994*. London: NCEPOD, 1996.
15. Masters RH, Cole JW, Walther AH, Flynn VJ, Prentiss RJ. Incidence of vascular accidents following transurethral prostatectomy. *J Urol* 1968; **100**: 544.
16. Roos NP, Wennberg JE, Malenka DJ *et al*. Mortality and reoperation after open and transurethral resection of the prostate for benign prostatic hyperplasia. *New Eng J Med* 1989; **320**: 1120.
17. Lu-Yao G, Barry MJ, Chang C-H, Wasson JH, Wennberg JE. Transurethral resection of the prostate among Medicare beneficiaries in the United States: time trends and outcomes. *Urology* 1994; **44**: 692.

18. Mebust WK. Increased mortality after transurethral prostatectomy for benign prostatic hyperplasia. *Curr Opinion Urol* 1992; **2**: 3.
19. Hargreave TB, Heynes CF, Kendrick SW, Whyte B, Clarke JA. Mortality after transurethral and open prostatectomy in Scotland. *Br J Urol* 1996; **77**: 547.
20. Holtgrewe HL. Prospective BPH Study. *AUA Today* 1990; 24.
21. Jenkins BJ, Sharma P, Badenoch DF, Fowler CG, Blandy JP. Ethics, logistics and a trial of transurethral versus open prostatectomy. *Br J Urol* 1992; **69**: 372.
22. Evans JWH, Singer M, Chapple CR *et al*. Haemodynamic evidence for perioperative cardiac stress during transurethral prostatectomy. *Br J Urol* 1991; **67**: 376.
23. Heyns CF, Rittoo D, Sutherland GR *et al*. Intraoperative myocardial ischaemia detected by biplane transoesophageal electrocardiography during transurethral prostatectomy. *Br J Urol* 1993; **71**: 5.
24. Lawson RA, Turner WH, Reeder MK, Sear JW, Smith JC. Haemodynamic effects of transurethral prostatectomy. *Br J Urol* 1993; **72**: 84.
25. Donovan J, Frankel S, Nanchahal K, Coast J, Williams M. *Prostatectomy for benign prostatic hyperplasia*. Bristol: Health Care Evaluation Unit, DHA, 1992.
26. Edwards LI, Lock R, Powell C, Jones P. Post-catheterization urethral strictures: a clinical and experimental study. *Br J Urol* 1983; **55**: 53.
27. Woodhouse E, Barnes R, Hadley H, Rothman C. Fibrous contracture of bladder neck. *Urology* 1979; **13**: 393.
28. Thorpe AC, Cleary R, Coles J *et al*. Deaths and complications following prostatectomy in 1404 men in the Northern Region of England: Northern Region Prostate Audit Group. *Br J Urol* 1994; **74**: 559.
29. Kaufman JJ. Incontinence after prostatectomy. In: Blandy JP, Lytton B (eds.) *The Prostate*. London: Butterworths, 1986: 71–81.
30. Gundian JC, Barrett DM, Parulkar BG. Mayo Clinic experience with the AS800 artificial urinary sphincter for urinary incontinence after transurethral resection of prostate or open prostatectomy. *Urology* 1993; **41**: 318.
31. Hanbury DC, Sethia KK. Erectile function following transurethral prostatectomy. *Br J Urol* 1995; **75**: 12.
32. Dunsmuir WD, Emberton M. There is significant sexual dysfunction following TURP. *Br J Urol* 1996; **77**: 39 (161) abstract.
33. Samdal F, Vada K, Lundmo P. Sexual function after transurethral prostatectomy. *Scand J Urol Nephrol* 1993; **27**: 27.
34. Thorpe AC, Cleary R, Coles J *et al*. Written consent about sexual function in men undergoing transurethral prostatectomy. *Br J Urol* 1994; **74**: 479.

Index